On qualifying, Dr Ellen Grant,
M.BCh.B (Commend),
D.Obst.R.C.O.G., began work first as a
research assistant and then as a clinical
assistant in the departments of Obstetrics
and Gynaecology and Endocrinology at
University College Hospital, London. It
was whilst she was working there that she
was asked to help with the London Trials
— the first major British study of the pill.
She has since worked for the FPA, the
Council for the Investigation of Fertility
Control and the Princess Margaret
Migraine Clinic at Charing Cross
Hospital. She is now a clinical ecologist in
private practice and is also an advisor to
Foresight (a charity concerned with pre-
conceptual care) and Action Against
Allergy, and is a member of both the
Council of the Dyslexia Institute and the
Committee of the City of London
Dyslexia Charity. She is the author of
several papers on the effects of the pill
that have appeared in the *British Medical
Journal* and the *Lancet*.

Dr Grant is married to a consultant
neurosurgeon and has a son and two
daughters. She lives in Surrey.

The Bitter Pill

How Safe is the 'Perfect Contraceptive'?

Dr Ellen Grant

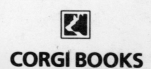

CORGI BOOKS

THE BITTER PILL
A CORGI BOOK 0 552 12798 1

Originally published in Great Britain by Elm Tree
Books/Hamish Hamilton Ltd.

PRINTING HISTORY
Elm Tree/Hamish Hamilton edition published 1985
Elm Tree/Hamish Hamilton edition reprinted 1985
Corgi edition published 1986

Copyright © 1985 by Dr Ellen Grant

This book is set in 10/11 pt Bodoni

Corgi Books are published by Transworld Publishers Ltd.,
61-63 Uxbridge Road, Ealing, London W5 5SA, in
Australia by Transworld Publishers (Aust.) Pty. Ltd., 26
Harley Crescent, Condell Park, NSW 2200, and in New
Zealand by Transworld Publishers (N.Z.) Ltd., Cnr.
Moselle and Waipareira Avenues, Henderson, Auckland.

Made and printed in Great Britain by
Cox & Wyman Ltd., Reading, Berks.

For my family and for everyone's family.

I have been told I should not write this book unless I had an alternative. It is a lifetime's work just trying to understand the problems. The search for something better belongs to us all.

Contents

Acknowledgements ix

1 Nature's Contraceptive? 13
2 The London Trials 22
   i) Hormone Balance 22
   ii) The Blood Clot Factor 33
   iii) Changes in the Brain 45
3 Swings and Roundabouts: Upsets in Metabolism 61
4 Even Worse than Smoking 68
5 Allergy, and How to Recover from the Pill 77
6 Trial and Error 103
7 Cancer and the Pill 115
8 What is Happening to the Young? 152
9 The Future Beckons 186

Appendices 203
Glossary 230
References 235
Useful Addresses 248
Index 250

Acknowledgements

I am very grateful for the invaluable support of my husband Norman and the help of many colleagues and friends who have contributed to my studies over the past twenty-five years. These include Dr Eleanor Mears, Dr John Pryse-Davies, Mrs Enid Vine, Mrs Barbara Lamb, Professor Merton Sandler, Dr Desmond Carroll, Dr Frank Clifford Rose, Mr Ian Burn, Dr Patricia Goodwin, Dr Tim Steiner, Dr Bruce Müller, Dr Bill Ollier, Professor Victor Wynn, Dr Gina Schoental, Dr Kitty Little, Dr Richard Mackarness, Dr John Mansfield, Dr George Lord, Professor Jack Pepys, Dr Ronald Finn, Dr Len McEwan, Dr John Howard, Professor Derek Bryce-Smith, Dr Stephen Davies and Dr Ifor Capel.

I should also especially like to thank Mrs Belinda Barnes of Foresight, Mrs Amelia Nathan Hill and Mrs Aeronwy Ellis of Action Against Allergy and Mrs Wendy Fisher and Dr Harry Chasty of the Dyslexia Institute and Dr Beve Hornsby of the Hornsby Centre for learning difficulties. Mrs Jean Robinson, ex-Chairman of the Patients' Association, gave advice on epidemiology, Mrs Jane Galbraith on statistics, Betty (EM) Thornton supplied key references and my collaborator Judy Kirby brought it all together. The typing load was carried by Mrs Audrey Condry, Mrs Yvonne Tralls, Deborah Goodall, and Judy Kirby. I should also like to thank my agent Deborah Rogers, Judith Hannam of Elm Tree Books and Emer O'Neill of Corgi Books.

The Bitter Pill

1 Nature's Contraceptive?

If the sixties were swinging, then the eighties are proving to be the decade when people want to be healthy. In twenty years our goal has changed from having fun to being fit and we have a growing suspicion of drugs, chemicals and conventional medicine. Yet one carry-over from the sixties is confounding this drive for healthier living and jeopardising future generations: the pill.

How can the modern young woman in her tracksuit square her desire for a balanced, healthy life with the lurking fear of damage to her body caused by steroid hormones? Can the older woman really believe that her menopause will become more normal if she takes horses' hormones? She cannot be reassured by the endless catalogue of medical research which is paraded before her in newspapers, magazines and on television. First a cancer scare, then a denial, then another juggle with hormone strengths to produce the safe dose — but try as they may, doctors cannot give the pill the full clearance women desire. As contradictions continue to emerge from research, the tone of advice is changing. We are now told that no drug can ever be free from side-effects, and the risks of cancer and vascular disease must be balanced against the problems of pregnancy, both social and medical. It is a subtle shifting of responsibility which means that women will ultimately have to accept that a price has to be paid for convenient contraception.

That something is going badly wrong must be apparent to any aware woman. Two screening practices have become household phrases in the past two years — breast self-examination and cervical smear tests. This is not just good health education in practice, these procedures are being promoted because of alarming increases in cancer of the breast and cervix, particularly in young women. The irony of this situation is that young women are being urged to examine their breasts while at the same time being prescribed a drug which can give them a breast disease, and advised to seek routine cervical smears because of a known link between their contraception and cancer. If prevention is the catchword of the eighties, it does not seem to be working here.

I took part in the first pill trials in London in 1961. I had been working as clinical assistant to Dr Gerald Swyer, consultant endocrinologist at University College Hospital, who was one of the first doctors in Britain to test the new hormones in women. I had heard of the revoluntionary method of birth control while studying at Dundee Medical School and realised at once how important this discovery was. The London Trials were carried out by the Council for the Investigation of Fertility Control and it was with a mixture of pride, ignorance, apprehension and the confidence of youth that I started my first ever clinic. The very next year the pill was available for British women. There was universal delight at the simplicity of it, but almost immediately the first serious side-effects, of venous thrombosis, were being reported in America and Britain.

At about this time my secretary at the clinic, who was taking the pill, collapsed with severe pain in her leg. She had suffered a thrombosis of her iliac artery, followed by paralytic ileus— paralysis of the gut muscle. This incident, however, did not distract me from my research. Like many doctors at that time, I thought such life-threatening events were unusual and if we tried enough different combinations the pill would be safe. Ten years later I realised this was not true and I stopped prescribing it. During those ten years I jockeyed with types and doses of the pill to prevent women suffering side-effects like migraine but by the late sixties I came to the conclusion that women with any kind of side-effect would be better off changing to a mechanical method of birth control. I became convinced that the two pill hormones would always cause too much illness and I believed that sooner or later the medical profession in general would agree.

The opposite has happened. We have experienced more than twenty years of unnecessary ill health in women and now a second generation of mothers and their children are being exposed to the harmful effects of steroid hormones. But what is more alarming is the fact that whereas in the sixties we were giving them to married women who had often completed their families, today younger and younger women are now going on the pill even though six studies[1] have found an increased risk of breast cancer from long-term use of oral contraceptives in women under twenty-five who had not yet had a baby. So far very few of these young women have been followed up in the large studies, but even from small numbers their increased risk is clear.

The pill, however, is a drug of such social and sexual convenience that its tragic consequences will continue to be disregarded until women fully realise the consequences of such convenience. Preferred ignorance has caused us to close our eyes to the enormous increase in ill health of young women since the pill was introduced and to the fact that the effects of the pill on allergies, vascular disease, mental health, cancer and congenital abnormalities are more powerful than the effects of smoking and show up in a much quicker time.

Everybody hopes that tomorrow a 'safer' pill will emerge and meanwhile optimistic researchers have tried to show us that the pill can confer protection from some diseases, such as benign breast lumps. But this is a case when statistics can distort the truth. In fact, the pill flushes out women with weak immune systems, producing early side-effects in them which persuade them to abandon it. A doctor may take a woman with breast lumps off the pill, or not allow one predisposed to them to take it in the first place.[2] In this way the women with the strongest immune systems are the ones who stay on the pill. The researchers study these women and declare that the pill has protected them from benign breast disease. The reality is that women who develop simple breast lumps stop the pill sooner than usual, while women who develop breast cancer have taken the pill for longer. The situation is further confused by the fact that whereas large doses of pill steroid can be used to suppress breast lumps, smaller doses like those in most pills can cause them to appear.

Once a drug has been used regularly over many years it almost becomes popular culture and it is as hard for doctors as it is for patients to abandon. Tranquillisers, which were introduced in the same decade as the pill, became the mainstay of many people who took them daily for up to twenty years. The recent backlash against them, plus economic pressure from the government, has persuaded GPs to prescribe less of these sedating drugs. And although they were always considered to be harmless and non-addictive, some of the long-term users discovered that they almost suffered the 'cold turkey' of narcotic addiction when they tried to withdraw.

With the constant stream of drug scares and drug-induced tragedies reported in the newspapers and the formation of organisations fighting for victim compensation, it is strange that the pill manages to resist unpopularity in our present anti-drug climate. For all our professed interest in fitness, do we in fact prize sexual freedom above health?

We were sitting in a bright, sunny lecture room in Dundee Medical School when we heard about the pill for the first time. Our lecturer told us that a revolutionary method of birth control, which worked by blocking brain hormones, had been developed in America and large scale trials had already begun in Puerto Rico. My first reaction was of wonder. Here was the magical solution to an age-old human dilemma — medicine put to the practical use of man. What I could not know then was the other side of this scientific success story, but at a time of discovery who questions the price?

The role of hormones in birth control, which sprang into the headlines so dramatically in the 1950s, was first noted in the nineteenth century when physiologists began to track down these chemical messengers. It became obvious to several researchers that a chemical agent was travelling via the blood-stream to communicate information and instruction to target organs. The tie-up with birth control came in the last part of the century when a crucial discovery was made. A researcher found that the secretions of a yellow coloured cyst in the ovary prevented the release of more eggs once a pregnancy had started. The substance had no name at that point and it was not until 1905 that the word 'hormone' — from the Greek 'I excite' — appeared on the scientific stage. Three years earlier a significant laboratory experiment in Britain had described how the pancreas produced digestive juices on instruction from the duodenum and the existence of the chemical messenger had been established. In 1921 (the year insulin was discovered), an Austrian doctor identified the yellow cyst secretions as hormones and declared they could be used as contraceptives. These *natural* hormones were later discovered to be *several types of oestrogen and one progesterone*.

The natural hormones our bodies make are unique to us. They are carefully and precisely made to suit our individual needs, moment by moment, and are monitored continuously by sensitive feedback mechanisms. We have them for regulating a number of bodily functions, including coping with stress. The sex hormones oestrogen and progesterone are made in our bodies from a fatty substance called cholesterol. However well laboratory manufactured hormones may chemically mimic our own home-grown brand they are still foreign substances and each of us may experience a different reaction to them. Evidence is accumulating now to show that women and children are becoming sensitive to their own hormones possibly as a result of the women taking oral contraceptives (*see* p. 170).

Once hormones had been 'discovered' manufacturers set

about producing them synthetically. The first approach had been to use animal sex hormones in women to mimic the high levels of pregnancy and prevent ovulation taking place. But animal production proved much too difficult and expensive to meet a demand which was being anticipated as universal. In 1928 the German firm Schering was the first to extract oestrogens from pigs' ovaries but they needed four tons from the sows just to get 25 milligrams of oestradiol! Later progesterone was extracted from the roots of a wild Mexican yam but this could not be taken orally as it is almost completely destroyed in the digestive tract. It is used today by injection and suppository to treat the premenstrual syndrome in an often mistaken belief that women suffering from period problems are short of progesterone.

The years before the first pill trials saw drug companies vying with each other to discover a cheap method of delivering hormones which could be taken by mouth. The revolutionary breakthrough came with the manufacture of *artificial testosterone*. Derivatives of this male hormone are present in nearly all of today's pills, although a few are derived from *artificial progesterone*. These are made in the laboratory from cholesterol derived from wool fat, cattle bile or plant steroids. Schering and the American firm Syntex were the first companies to produce these orally active hormones mimicking progesterone. In Europe the drugs became known as progestogens and in America, progestins. *These steroids are between 1000 and 5000 times more powerful than natural progesterone*.

Animals reacted in a wide variety of ways when given the new hormone preparations. There were changes in their carbohydrate, fat and protein metabolism, and alterations in their salt and water balance. Male or female hormone effects could be blocked or stimulated and the actions of several brain hormones were blocked. Given during pregnancy, animals sometimes produced offspring with abnormalities. Later I was to write, with my colleague Dr Eleanor Mears, to the *British Medical Journal*[3] to declare that the effect in women 'is not necessarily the same as the effect in animals'. We were too optimistic. The animal tests proved to be excellent predictors of the effects in humans, especially their ability to cause cancer.

It was no new discovery that oestrogens given to experimental animals caused breast cancer by stimulating rapid cell growth — it was known in 1932. But in spite of this most oral contraceptives today are a mixture of oestrogens and progestogens. The original pill trials in America used progestins only because of the cancer risk but the first ones tested clinically by Dr John Rock, a Harvard gynaecologist, were impure and contained some oestrogen. And when 'pure' progestins were given, women complained of too much bleeding. It was then realised that for good cycle control a progestin needed the addition of an oestrogen.

Dr Rock and Dr Gregory Pincus tried out the first combined pill in the fifties on a Harvard volunteer group and on some chronic mentally ill patients. Both men and women took an early form of Enovid (10mg), which successfully stopped ovulation in the women and halted sperm production in the men. But the men were soon wheeled out of these trials when one of them displayed shrunken testicles, visible proof of something going wrong.

The 'male pill' seems to have floundered at this hurdle. But later on even the unexplained deaths of three women in Puerto Rico who were in the pill trials did not seriously hamper progress.[4] By then millions of women world-wide were taking part in the greatest mass pill experiment in history and the spectre of overpopulation was thought to be finally on the run.

How Women's Sex Hormones Work

* A woman is born with a lifetime's supply of eggs in her ovaries, which lie in the pelvis on either side of the womb. They are controlled by a biological 'clock' which can tick happily away for as long as forty years. The clock, sited in the hypothalamus and pituitary gland at the base of the brain, sends out chemical messengers, hormones, to stimulate the development and the release of eggs. The brain hormones also control the secretion of oestrogens and progesterone from the ovary.

* In the first half of the menstrual cycle, the pituitary's follicle stimulating hormone (FSH) develops an egg while its protective cyst secretes oestrogens. The oestrogen production falls just before ovulation, and the egg bursts out of its protective cyst. The ruptured cyst turns yellow and is known as the corpus luteum. It now secretes progesterone as well as several oestrogens. Progesterone simply means 'a steroid which prepares for pregnancy', and its production is stimulated by the pituitary's luteinising hormone (LH).

* Oestrogens thicken the lining of the womb after the previous month's growth has been shed during the monthly bleeding. Oestrogen also stimulates the cells lining the glands to grow rapidly, divide and proliferate.

* After ovulation progesterone instructs these cells to secrete a mixture of starch and protein, hopefully to feed a new life. Together these hormones are responsible for enlarging the blood vessels to bring in more blood and to form the placenta.

* In pregnancy, an egg is propelled along a fallopian tube until it meets sperm swimming towards it. One sperm usually penetrates one egg which starts to divide into a mass of cells and then embeds, a few days later, into the womb wall. Levels of the sex hormones oestrogen and progesterone rise and egg production stops.

* The hormone levels go on rising during pregnancy and because of their high profile in the body the brain stops

secreting its egg stimulating hormones. This is the action that synthetic hormones mimic, continually duping the brain into believing that pregnancy has occurred.

* In pregnancy, the developing embryo produces a hormone called 'hGG', which stimulates increasing secretion of oestrogen and progesterone from the corpus luteum during the first three months. Then the placenta takes over hormone production until the baby signals that it is ready to be born almost exactly nine months from the first day of the last menstrual period. More progesterone is converted to oestrogen, making the progesterone levels fall suddenly. As oestrogen production increases, labour pains are felt and the baby is born a few hours later.

* The pill causes medical castration. Normal menstrual cycles and normal hormone production ceases. A woman does not usually have painful periods when she is on the pill because she does not ovulate.

* Two days after the pills are stopped the withrawal of these hormones induces a scanty bleeding. A woman on the pill does not have normal periods.

* See page 226 for a list of hormone preparations.

2   The London Trials

(i) Hormone Balance — No Room to Manoeuvre

Common belief: *Each woman can have a pill to suit her individual hormone balance.*

Fact: *Commonly used pills have an almost identical hormone balance.*

The prospect of an overcrowded planet was the initial spur to find a simple, foolproof method to control the feared population explosion. The pill may have been welcomed by middle-class couples everywhere but the original research was done with the Third World more in mind. In America the money needed to test oral contraceptives was raised by the veteran women's rights campaigner Margaret Sanger and her involvement has nurtured the myth that the pill is part of women's liberation.

My introduction to the revolution in birth control came in 1961 when I was twenty-six and working as a clinical assistant to Dr Gerald Swyer, a consultant endocrinologist at University College Hospital, London. He and Dr Gregory Pincus were the co-chairmen of the Oral Contraceptive Advisory Group to the International Planned Parenthood Federation. This was a prestigious group made up of fifty international doctor-scientists, but only six of them were women. I was asked whether I would like to test the new contraceptive pill for the Family Planning Association. The job meant consulant pay only two years after qualifying as a doctor — it was an excellent offer.

There were other reasons why I accepted immediately. From earliest memories of childhood I had understood that there was no more serious problem in the world than over-population. I remember my Scottish father spelling out the consequences of too many people — wars, poverty, starvation, pollution. He felt strongly about this threat to civilisation and over the years communicated this concern to me. I was therefore extremely pleased to be asked to take part in the first pill trials in London.

In America, Mexico and Puerto Rico, large doses of both hormones were given as combined pills in the fifties and sixties trials. Although there has always been a high dis-continuation rate with any type of pill, large doses are surprisingly well tolerated. They mimic the high hormone levels in the last six months of pregnancy when women often feel well and look happy. Nausea was a common complaint with them, however, and the other main problem was too much pituitary suppression with no withdrawal bleeding (amenorrhoea). In order to combat this, they tested several pills, cutting the doses in half each time.

In London the aim was to seek the lowest dose possible which did not allow ovulation. Women today are under the impression that the search for a low dose pill is a recent investigation but this is precisely what we were doing in the London Trials in the sixties. My early work has often been dismissed in the mistaken belief that I have been only talking about high doses of progestogens. Yet all commonly used pills must have a high enough dose of progestogen otherwise there will be break-through bleeding. The recent attempts to use the weaker, low dose pills — which we discarded in the sixties — have resulted in more pregnancies when the pill cycle has been interrupted or when antibiotics have been taken for an infection. Women are more likely to conceive on these 'safer' pills and that's why we discarded them. Although we wanted to identify the pills with the best hormone balance which would produce the fewest side-effects for British women, the real aim of the London Trials was to find the lowest doses which would prevent pregnancy.

Dr Eleanor Mears, the FPA's medical secretary, had

already been testing the hormones in a small number of patients. She was a first-class organiser. She had the trial forms ready for me to use and offered to take over clinics if my baby son became ill. Feeling reassured by this support, I began my task with great enthusiasm.

There was plenty of enthusiasm in FPA circles in those days, it was infectious. The few doctors who were prescribing the pill were in demand as lecturers at clinics all over the country with their stories of delighted women patients whose sex lives had been made simple at last. The reaction of one woman who told me 'my husband brings me flowers now' was typical. If women loved the simplicity of the method, doctors saw an end to the troublesome climb in world population. But while they waited in anticipation of the development taking off nationally, Dr Mears and I had to deal with more immediate problems.

Our study involved thousands of women in London, and later in York, Edinburgh, Liverpool, Birmingham, Newcastle and Glasgow. There were seven progestogens and two oestrogens in manufacture then and we were testing three types:

1) combined, where two hormones are given together in one pill for twenty or twenty-one days followed by a gap of seven days;
2) sequential pills, usually oestrogen for twenty days with a progestogen added on the last five days followed by a gap of seven;
3) progestogen only, when a pill is taken every day.

Each of the drug companies involved donated both the pills and funds to the Council for the clinical testing of the different products, unlike in America where each research centre tended to be financed by one large company. Women volunteers were enrolled at the London FPA headquarters. They were married women aged between twenty-five and forty-four, healthy, of normal weight, and of proven higher fertility than average. Research work in America had found that only one out of three couples achieve a pregnancy within two months but our ladies had a far higher score — nine out of ten had quickly become pregnant and in fact half of them had already had accidental pregnancies. Nevertheless, they agreed to run the risk of further accidental pregnancies as they calculated that this risk was less with the pill than other methods — a view which turned out to be a little misplaced when several women later became pregnant on the lower dose pills.

My role was to take a careful history from each woman and give her a thorough examination, weight and blood pressure checks, and a test for anaemia. I sent vaginal and cervical smears and small samples from the lining of the womb to pathologists every six months.

Control groups of women — those using an alternative method such as the cap — were not enrolled in the early trials. Normally in double blind studies, two groups are monitored at the same time, but oral contraceptives were a different case. If a new hay fever tablet is being tested, for example, half the volunteers would be given dummy pills — not a practice which could be used with women requiring contraceptive protection. In those days women generally paid for their caps, creams, pessaries and sheaths from the FPA and the only people getting free birth control were the trial volunteers. As the drug companies were paying for the testing to be done it was no doubt thought improper to ask them to pay up for mechanical methods in order to include a control group in the trials. At the time, however, it was not seen as an impediment on the trials as the purpose was to find the pills most acceptable to the majority of women. It was only in the late sixties when the NHS started paying for contraception that full controlled trials were done.

We eventually tried out over seventy different combinations of two oestrogens and seven progestogens, and it was particularly satisfactory to find that none of our very fertile volunteers became pregnant when taking the first pill we tested. But there were some disturbing trends developing.

Side-Effects

Although breakthrough bleeding while the volunteers were on the pills was being faithfully recorded at all the trial centres, the side-effects appeared to be more arbitrarily reported. Side-effects only seemed to be noted when the doctor concerned remembered to ask specific questions about headaches, depression or anxiety. Many doctors feel it is important that women should not be encouraged to imagine 'neurotic' symptoms. There is a tendency to dismiss women's various complaints as biased. Often women were not asked directly about possible symptoms as this might put the idea into their heads.

While we were preparing to add some of the unpleasant effects women told me of to our first published results we were told that we were emphasising the negative aspects of the drug when its benefits were overwhelming. Our first report in the *British Medical Journal* in 1962[1] showed that none of the 100 volunteers had become pregnant, their periods were regular with withdrawal bleeding happening two days after the pills were stopped, bleeding was lighter, they had less cramps and premenstrual tension, and breasts were less tender for some women. Cycle control was excellent with only two in a hundred cases of breakthrough bleeding. But the other side to the story was that women were also complaining of full-blown classical migraine, of loss of interest in love-making, of depression. The complaints of migraine, sometimes experienced for the first time, were increasing. One woman who was desperate to limit her family tried four different preparations but always finished up bedridden with such severe migraine that the neighbours had to take care of the children. In my experience, people do not imagine the symptoms of classical migraine, with its vision impairment, pain and nausea.

What Was Happening?

I was very interested in finding physical reasons for the side-effects being reported to me. I had an unrewarding experience attending seminars dealing with psycho-sexual counselling, which Dr Mears thought might help me handle women complaining of loss of libido. She suggested to me that although some women taking the pill might well lose interest in sex, there could be a psychological component. They may have been pinning their hopes on the pill for resolving some sexual difficulty and when they were disappointed in this invented a side-effect to put the blame on. In my view this was not an argument which fitted the facts. What was behind the huge swings in mood caused by the different pills, the weight gain in some women, the headaches and depression? Luck had provided me with the best tool then available to investigate these differences — my microscope.

Scientists who work with animals — whom I would meet at yearly gatherings of the Society for the Study of Fertility — don't usually offer psychological excuses for animal behaviour although animals can react to excess stress just like humans. But was it possible to measure physical changes to prove that my patients were not neurotic? That was what I wanted to do. The opportunity luckily presented itself when the pathologist handling the endometrial biopsies on the trials decided to emigrate and I was offered the job. This gave me the chance to see under a microscope what effect the pill was having on the womb.

Exciting Discoveries

I was able to examine the biopsy slides at home while my son went to nursery school and his baby sister slept outside in her pram. Not long after I had become used to the appearances of the womb lining on the different days of the normal cycle and had begun to catalogue the changes caused by the different pills, I made an exciting discovery. One sample had thin scanty tissue typical of the effect of a progestogen but there was also a large group of thick-walled small arteries, called arterioles. The woman whose sample this was had been in the clinic complaining of severe migraine attacks, depression and loss of libido. Her pre-pill biopsy sample had appeared normal, with large glands and only a small group of arterioles. Now she had such prominent arterioles in her womb that I wondered if there was any connection with the fact that on this pill she was having migraine attacks. I remembered seeing in reports from Dr Edris Rice-Wray in Mexico that some women had strange vascular patterns in their endometrium. I was convinced there was a connection. We gave this woman a different pill, one with four times less progestogen but the same dose of oestrogen as the pill she had been on. She became less depressed and her migraine stopped.

But now she had sore leg veins and dizziness. Her endometrial sample showed no arteriole groups — instead, dilated small veins. I wondered whether this meant that endometrial vessels were not only reflecting changes in the arteries of the head but also in the veins throughout the body.

By this time I had found that more and more women with thick groups of endometrial arterioles also had headaches or migraine. Why these women should have vessels which seem to be more numerous and grow more thickly than those of other women in response to hormone stimulation is a puzzle still not resolved today. Dr Kitty Little, an Oxford scientist, later was to write that the male derivatives in the pill, the nor-testosterones, developed animals' blood vessels so that they became thicker and more irregular than usual. What was obvious, however, was that some women were more susceptible than others. I looked back at 200 pre-pill biopsy samples of our volunteers' normal cycles and found that some had more groups of arterioles in the earlier parts of their menstrual cycles. These were the women more likely to get headaches.[2]

Hormone Balance and Headaches

Of the first 500 women enrolled with us, 10 per cent had headaches before they started the pill, usually just before or during a period, and at other times of hormone stress like puberty, childbirth or even while under mental and physical stress. A smaller percentage reported having migraine. These two groups tended to get bad headaches with any pill but we then discovered that some of the pill combinations gave migraine to as many as six women out of ten within their first twelve pill cycles — some experienced it for the first time in their lives. Not all pills had this effect. Some caused headaches in only one out of ten women and some volunteers even ceased having headaches. One pill, containing the highest doses of both oestrogen and progestogen, prevented such premenstrual symptoms in nearly everyone. High doses of steroids were suppressing headaches and mood changes but were also more likely to cause amenorrhoea — no withdrawal bleeding at all.

During the shuffling around of doses we came to realise that it was not the high or low doses of progestogen which caused the most headaches but the middle range when combined with the same dose of oestrogen. We found that there was a *peak dose* combination for headaches. We tested three doses of oestrogen with the same dose of progestogen and again it was the middle amount which was the culprit. The combined pills were causing more headaches than oestrogen or progestogen used singly. But that was the rub, the single dose pills had disadvantages of their own — especially irregular bleeding and unplanned pregnancies.

The conclusion I came to was that proportion was the key. A change as small as 15 micrograms of oestrogen or half a milligram of progestogen can mean the difference between a pill which causes a lot of headaches or very few.[3]

Hormones and headache seem to go together in the normal cycle. There is a fall in blood oestrogen at ovulation and again just before a period. These are the times women can experience headaches although the premenstrual phase seems to create more. Blood vessels become more sensitive to biochemical changes then because they are developed and altered by cyclical hormones. As it happens, *it is the same chemicals which control both our blood vessel reactions and our moods and behaviour*. These chemicals are also altered by hormone changes and diet and they become more likely to pass through the barrier from the blood into the brain tissues at period times. This explains why women sometimes get headache premenstrually if they eat cheese, chocolate or oranges or drink alcohol, when at other times of the month they eat them without suffering.

An Australian neurologist[4] who studied women with migraine found that oestrogen and progesterone levels in their blood varied widely before periods. Their migraines came on when oestrogen levels fell even though their progestrone production was still up. This was an interesting study and contradicts the fashionable treatment of the premenstrual syndrome with progesterone given in the often mistaken belief that all sufferers lack progesterone, although some women do have a fall in progesterone before their oestrogen levels drop. The suppression of symptoms by massive doses of steroids may give a temporary benefit.[5] But I have seen many women whose symptoms and allergic reactions become extremely severe after so-called natural progesterone therapy. Such premenstrual tension treatment induced an early menopause in a doctor's wife of thirty-five. A year later she still feels ill and extremely angry that she was prescribed such a drastic remedy.

At the beginning of the London Trials we tried endlessly to find the right dose combinations to stop the women volunteers having side-effects. Headaches affected up to 60 per cent of women within a year of taking those progestogenic pills which had a prolonged late secretory effect and marked development of endometrial arterioles. But when I brought up the matter of the headaches and migraine — which I considered to be an early warning sign — at a Council meeting when a pill's future marketing was being discussed, the reaction of members stunned me. There was utter silence. This silence, heard at so many medical gatherings since, seems to have grown into a deafening roar.

By now we knew very well that although it was easy to prevent headaches by changing the pill doses we tended to run into other problems.

In 1964[6] I published a method for estimating the hormone balance of a pill by studying the womb changes. In the months before starting the pill, samples of endometrium from 200 women showed growth in the first half of the cycle. Secretion appeared under the cell nucleus (subnuclear vacuoles) between days sixteen and eighteen, a sign that the women had ovulated and were now making progesterone. The womb lining continued to grow and the secretion emptied into the large glands ready to feed a fertilised embryo. In the last few days of the cycle the womb vessels enlarged and dilated.

It was quite different when the women were taking a combined progestogen pill. I could hardly find any tissue as there had been very little growth. The lining was very thin with a few small glands scattered around. As the pills were started on day five of the cycle I could see secretion within two or three days but then there was little activity for the rest of the cycle. But some women had surprisingly large blood vessels as I have just described.

By contrast, the sequential pills where oestrogen was given for ten or fifteen days before progestogen was added, caused a thick overgrowth of glands and tissues.

31

I worked out that if secretion appeared on days seven to eleven that pill would give women regular cycles. In about ninety-six cycles out of 100 they would have a withdrawal bleeding within two days of stopping their pills. When I saw the secretions (vacuoles) for most of the pill cycle, the women were likely to bleed before they had taken their twenty pills. For example, if a pill showed vacuoles from days ten or twenty the women would bleed early in nearly half of their cycles. If a pill was neither mainly acting like an oestrogen or mainly acting like a progestogen, women were more likely to bleed early. The *weaker* progestogen pills not only caused unexpected bleeding, which was sometimes heavy, but also *failed to prevent ovulation and unplanned pregnancies*, as did the sequentials containing less than 0.1mg mestranol. *For this reason nearly all pills used now are mostly progestogenic in their actions.* [7]

In 1969 we tested four progestogen-only pills in Yugoslavia. [8] With megestrol acetate 0.25mg nearly half the women became pregnant while chlormadinone 0.5mg and norethisterone acetate 0.3mg and norgestrel 0.05mg gave pregnancy rates of 12, 4 and 9 per 100 women years respectively. None of them as good as the combined pill. Although the dose of 0.25mg had been too low to change the endometrium, it did alter the cervical mucus — an early clue that the cervix might be especially sensitive to the carcinogenic efforts of progestogens as was already being discovered by Professor Weid and Dr Melamed in America (*see* p. 118).

By the latter part of the sixties I had calculated that when you vary the hormone balance of a pill and increase the progestogen strength you change the side-effects from irregular bleeding to distended veins, to irritability, weight gain and artery changes, to depression and loss of libido.

Summary

* Pills containing:
  high progestogen and high oestrogen cause amenorrhoea (no bleeding)
  high progestogen and low oestrogen cause regular scanty withdrawal bleeding
  low progestogen and low oestrogen cause irregular bleeding and pregnancy risk
  low progestogen and high oestrogen cause vein changes

* Sequential pills (like regime used in hormone replacement therapy) lead to overgrowth of the lining of the womb

* Occurrence of headache and thickened arteries with the first 12 cycles from 1 up to 6 out of 10 women taking different pills

* First year discontinuation rate is high among sensitive women taking pills which cause either headaches or breakthrough bleeding

(ii) The Blood Clot Factor

Common belief: *Thrombosis is only a risk with high dose oestrogen pills.*

Fact: *Serious changes in arteries and veins can happen with any pill in susceptible women.*

The most striking effect of the pill is the variation in *individual* susceptibility. Different pills do different things to different women. Some women have severe and disabling reactions to any type of pill while others escape symptoms for years.

The switching of symptoms with a changeover of pill is hardly surprising, as both hormones alter amine metabolism which controls blood vessel reactivity, and mood and behaviour. In our studies in the sixties we found small variations in dose of either oestrogen or progestogen could vary side-effects, and changes in blood vessels and enzymes. Each new dose would simply throw up another side-effect in some other bodily function.

The most 'notorious' side-effect in the early days was thrombosis. Since it was a startling and sometimes fatal consequence, it gained the best newspaper and television coverage. One of the first cases was described in the *Lancet*[1] by a Suffolk GP whose patient, a nurse, had suffered a clot in both lungs. Thrombosis simply means a blood clot. Clots can form in either arteries or veins and clog up the blood circulation. Clots can cause strokes, paralysis, heart attacks or severe abdominal pain. A common site for clots is the leg veins and this is a potentially dangerous condition because the clot can travel up to the lungs. Sudden damage to the lungs is as much an instant death sentence as a heart attack.

Thrombosis may be one of the commonest causes of death for the elderly but is rare in the young. This may have accounted for the publicity although in fact cancer kills twice as many women who have taken the pill. Increased risk of thrombosis occurs when there are changes in blood, blood flow and vessel walls. Amongst pill takers we found that vein complaints were most likely with either oestrogen or progestogen pills which had either a higher dose or balance of oestrogen and especially if they dilated the endometrial sinusoids.[2]

We were in a unique position in London. Almost alone we were able to investigate a very wide range of doses. Not all of these were eventually put on the market and very few had been given a 'trade' name at this stage. Soon we had looked at six doses of norgestrol, five doses of ethynodiol diacetate, four doses of norethisterone acetate and three doses of norethisterone. Some of the lower doses which were then rejected were later marketed as low-dose pills and are still being widely used.

Distended Veins

As we swapped women from higher to lower dose pills more and more women began to complain of sore legs instead of headaches. Some developed masses of tiny twisting veins just below the skin. Others showed distended, painful varicose veins. Some volunteers found their ankles had begun to swell while others complained of haemorrhoids. Several women developed superficial thrombophlebitis — an inflamed clotting of the surface veins, while a few suffered from threateningly large clots in the deeper veins. Some were admitted to hospital with severe a abdominal pains, possibly because of thrombosis in the blood vessels of the gut. Others were hospitalised for a condition like meningitis with severe headaches and neck stiffness, but with no sign of infection. These mysterious illnesses were becoming too common. We seemed to be running into more trouble more quickly with the pills that had lower doses of progestogen. Many of these low dose pills, especially those with 0.1mg of mestranol were soon withdrawn from testing and not put on the market.

Instead of thick groups of little arteries I was now seeing dilated endometrial sinusoids whether or not the pill had an overall progestogen or oestrogen action. Eventually I calculated that it was the pills with a higher dose or balance of oestrogen which were dilating the veins, but either oestrogen alone or a progestogen alone did not cause such severe changes. Once more it was a peak combination of the two hormones that did the damage. By now the peak effects were happening at different doses and beginning to look like a range of mountains. Using the microscope I could predict what was likely to happen to the women.

Mrs M was very nervous and tight when I first examined her. After six months on a pill with a high dose of oestrogen and progestogen (norethisterone 2mg plus mestranol 0.1mg) she felt relaxed and confessed she was enjoying sexual intercourse for the first time. The sample from her womb showed the typical small inactive glands of a progestogen with tiny veins among swollen tissue cells. After two years the veins were more dilated and by three years there was a thickening of tissue cells around their thin walls. One year later I was sent a sample from Mrs M's clinic. I remember being shocked to see a sinusoid so large that it nearly filled the whole microscopic field. I telephoned the clinic to find out what had happened to Mrs M. After 40 cycles on the pill she had complained of migraine for the first time in her life and during cycle 43 she developed thrombophlebitis — not just in one leg but in both and at the same time. The clinic doctor had already given the advice to stop taking the pill.

Most pill research and publicity has focused on oestrogens increasing blood clotting but there is very little awareness, even among the medical profession, that it is the combined pills that cause the most dramatic changes in the blood vessels themselves. It is hardly ever mentioned that combinations of both hormones cause rapid growth and distortion of blood vessels. These changes have been found all over the body in susceptible women. The most severely affected blood vessels are those of the target organs, the womb and the ovaries, threatening a woman's future fertility.

Blood Changes

Our blood contains its own rescue system to prevent loss through injury. When we bleed after a cut it should soon coagulate because of the presence of cells called platelets. The stickiness of these cells, which effectively 'plug' the cut, is caused by a clotting factor which produces threads of fibrin.

Clotting factors are increased during pregnancy due to the high oestrogen levels so of course the pills with oestrogen do the same, with one important exception. The fail-safe anti-thrombin III, which prevents clotting, is decreased by the pill.

Clotting diseases are unusual in a normal pregnancy but the risk of thrombosis and pulmonary embolism is greater just after the baby is born when oestrogen drugs are given to stop lactation. There are two other events when the risk is higher — after a surgical operation or in cancer patients.

Dr Helen Payling Wright, who discovered the sticky platelets, found that the platelets of new mothers increased in number and stickiness each day after delivery until the tenth day, and then they began to lose the stickiness.[3] The risk to a woman after childbirth occurs on the day there are most sticky platelets — and this risk is increased three times if oestrogens are given. Women on the pill have larger numbers of sticky platelets than is usual.

I learned more about platelets from Dr Kitty Little in Oxford who has spent many years investigating the effects of steroids on bone marrow.[4] The red and white cells and the platelets are produced in the bone marrow. Giant cells called megakaryocytes are responsible for the tiny platelets, and one of the effects of the combined pill on the marrow is to distort these developing cells which leads to a greatly increased production of abnormally sticky platelets. In experiments, masses of tiny clots were found in the bones, liver, spleen and kidneys in rabbits.

Blood Flow Changes

Volunteers complained to me of leg cramps and distended painful veins which woke them in the night. Under the microscope the sore veins could be seen as dilated sinusoids and the women with cramps displayed a thickening of cells round the walls of the sinusoids, a condition called 'stromal condensation'. I wondered whether this thickening was being reflected in the calf muscles, where the waste products of cell metabolism may have been trapped in tiny veins instead of entering the bloodstream. If so, the night cramps could be explained because during rest waste products accumulate whereas movement speeds up circulation.

We had twelve women who developed superficial venous phlebitis or deep venous thrombosis after one year on the pill, and leg cramps had been among their complaints. The length of time on any pill seemed to increase the likelihood of dilated sinusoids and serious vascular accidents. It soon seemed a good idea to get women with cramps off the pill they were taking.

Vessel Wall Changes

In 1970[5] three Washington DC army pathologists studied the blood vessels of twenty young women who died while taking oral contraceptives. Although by that date there had been detailed clinical reporting of thrombosis in pill takers, there was little attention paid to the pathological findings.

Only nine of the women in the army doctors' study were known to be taking the pill as a contraceptive. Five were prescribed it for 'medical' reasons, painful periods, heavy or irregular bleeding. The shortest time of pill taking was five weeks and the longest thirteen months. Most had taken the pill for less than six months and most were in their twenties, the youngest was only eighteen. Some had been taking tranquillisers, one took cortisone and two were on thyroid extract.

Still recent clots were found in vessels *all over the body* including the lung, liver, abdomen and legs. Most of the vessels had thickened patches in the inner layers of the artery and vein walls — sometimes nearly filling the entire vessel. Two of the women had uterine fibroids — common with the pills — and one had hyperplastic breast disease. Three had chronic inflammation of the cervix. One had sudden blindness due to an arterial thrombosis. Another two had nobbly arteries and localised thickening of all three layers of the pulmonary artery — something unusual in non-pill users. One of these women was not known to have been on the pill and had been chosen as a control but it was later discovered that she had taken an oral contraceptive for six weeks before her death. These irregular changes in the artery wall indicate a more turbulent or stagnant blood flow making haemorrhage or thrombosis more likely.

Although I had already described that arterial thickening affected up to six out of ten women within a year of taking some oral contraceptives, one of the army pathologists wrote that these are *rare* individuals whose vascular tissues reacted to sex steroids in an idiosyncratic fashion so that the thickening would gradually close up major vessels. This statement was investigated further by US Air Force gynaecologists in 1977.[6] They examined the main artery to the womb taken from women having hysterectomies. Nearly all of the forty-four patients who had taken combined pills, or so-called 'natural oestrogens' or medroxy progesterone (one case only), had moderate to severe thickening of the inner layer of their arteries. The seven women who had never taken hormones before their hysterectomies did not have such changes. Most of the pill takers had used the pill for less than five years, but those who had taken the pill for longer had more severely affected vessels. Most had stopped the pill several years before. These changes did not relate to hypertension or smoking. Two of the conjugated oestrogen users had cancer of the endometrium.

The increased risk of haemorrhage in the tissues round the brain has been estimated as six times for pill users and twenty-two times for pill users who also smoke. Weak areas in blood vessels may be present from birth and can form a sac known as an aneurysm but the situation is aggravated by the pill and neuro-surgeons have become used to operating on young women who have bled from aneurysms (subarachnoid haemorrhages) after taking oral contraceptives.

The pill is also likely to cause hardening of the arteries due to the fact that it causes high blood pressure. Pills which cause a lot of headaches and artery changes in the womb vessels are especially likely to cause high blood pressure. The longer a woman takes even a low dose pill, the greater her chance of developing high blood pressure. The hormones controlling the blood pressure are altered by the pill and vessel damage in the kidneys can in turn cause more rises in blood pressure. Tiny clots in the kidneys' blood supply cause dead areas and scarring which cause a reflex rise in blood pressure raising chemicals. Another cause of high blood pressure is kidney damage from infections. Urinary infections are much more likely to become chronic in pill takers and repeated attacks cause kidney damage. Many women who need kidney transplants could have had their kidneys damaged by taking the pill.

In 1969 I published the Council for the Investigation of Fertility Control trial vein thrombosis results. We had seen 12 cases in 797 new patients completing 16,892 cycles, which equals 9 per 1,000 women per year. But for those women who took a low progestogen, high oestrogen pill (174 women completing 3,027 cycles) the rate was 26 per 1,000 per year. The weak progestogen pills with the big dose of mestranol gave us significantly more complaints of sore legs and cramps.

Dose Change

At about the same time the high oestrogen pills were dealt a mortal blow. The Committee on Safety of Drugs (now the Committee on Safety of Medicines) gathered evidence which was accepted as proof that thrombosis was more likely with a high dose of oestrogen.[7] Until then I had been led to believe that, as mestranol is converted in the body to ethinyl oestradiol, mestranol 0.1mg was equal in strength to ethinyl oestradiol 0.05mg but overnight, any pill containing more than 0.05mg oestrogen was withdrawn from use as a contraceptive, although the evidence was not published until the next year.[8]

Doctors voluntarily sent the CSD yellow cards detailing side-effects and in the early days most of these tended to come from the two FPA centres in London and Edinburgh. Few doctors seemed to be bothering with these except us, so our side-effect reports represented the tip of the iceberg.

The CSD evidence had another flaw. While I had undoubtedly found more thrombosis with some higher oestrogen pills there was also another explanation. On average, our volunteers had taken high dose pills for twice as long as low oestrogen pills. Women were able to tolerate these pills for longer because they need enough oestrogen to make them happy — the lower doses made them miserable — and thrombosis usually takes longer than twelve months to appear. The moves to a lower dose of oestrogen did not really improve the overall picture. Taking pills with more than 0.05mg off the market might reduce vein complaints by a third, but headaches and mood changes would be increased. I found that among 341 women stopping different pills because of side-effects the percentages were:

	Headache syndrome %	Mood changes %	Vein changes %
Combined pills			
High dose oestrogen	30	30	30
Low dose oestrogen	50	45	22
Sequentials	56	34	24

Sweden also reduced the oestrogen in pills in 1968 and by 1980 the incidence of venous thromboembolic disease had fallen by 30 per cent, but there was no improvement on the incidence of arterial complications or mortality rates.[9]

It is difficult for individual specialists[10] to be aware of the true incidence of serious side-effects. The commonly held view is that severe side-effects are rare, after all only a tiny proportion of cases are ever reported in the world's medical press. However, in America in the early sixties although only a few cases of thrombosis were initially recorded, when newspapers carried the story of this side-effect, the number of cases reported increased in dramatic fashion. True incidence is often much greater than the recorded number and the fact that the third patient we enrolled in 1961 developed a brain haemorrhage and thrombosis and the twelfth patient developed benign intracranial hypertension casts doubt on the belief that serious side-effects are rare.

Mrs C was very grateful to be our third patient enrolled in 1961. She had a large family and a difficult husband, so she was delighted to be free from the fears of yet another pregnancy. She was in her late thirties and her blood pressure was 140/90, which is borderline for being hypertensive, when I checked her four years after she started the pill. She then attended another clinic and when I next saw her two years later I was shocked to find her blood pressure had rocketed to 210/140. She had gained about 20lb and was complaining of tiredness, depression, irritability and headaches. She also had an enlarged womb, probably due to fibroids. I referred her to a gynaecologist for a hysterectomy, telling her she would not need to take the pill afterwards.

Unfortunately, she did not wish to have an operation and went on taking the pills she had accumulated over the years. Six months later she was suddenly rushed to Guy's Hospital with a brain haemorrhage. The neurosurgeon removed a blood clot, but the pathologist discovered that the haemorrhage had followed a cerebral artery thrombosis. The vessels in the brain at operation showed thickening without atheroma and necrotic areas and thrombi — changes very similar to those in the womb vessels.

The sad postscript to this story was that although Mrs C made a good recovery, she had a right-sided paralysis and slurred speech. She telephoned me and, with difficulty, asked if she could have some more pills. It is a tragedy to think that some women are too frightened to stop taking the pill, even when they know it is making them ill. This does not apply to married women so much today, but unmarried women are still scared to stop the pill.

In 1965 Dr Frank Walsh in Baltimore reviewed the international literature of sixty-three cases which involved brain or eye complications among pill takers.[11] The brain syndromes included twenty-five strokes, mostly due to artery or brain thrombosis. There were four cases of benign intracranial hypertension and another developed with a sixth nerve paralysis one month after the steroids had been discontinued. In our trial we too had had one diagnosed case of benign intracranial hypertension. She was the twelfth patient enrolled in 1961. Mrs JR gained 28lb in weight after seventy cycles on the pill and she was admitted to the Atkinson Morley neurosurgical hospital because of headaches and visual disturbances. She had raised pressure in the brain ventricles and papilloedema (swollen vessels in the back of the eye). Benign intracranial hypertension is known to occur when steroids such as cortisone or prednisone are withdrawn but can also occur when steroids like the pill are being taken.

Dr Walsh found the eye symptoms were mostly caused by artery or vein thrombosis and also by vasculitis. There were eight cases of optic neuritis. This is usually an early sign of a demyelinating disease know as multiple sclerosis (MS) and two cases did develop widespread symptoms. One of the women developed loss of vision one month after starting norethynodrel and mestranol for menorrhagia (heavy periods) and was later diagnosed as suffering from a 'fulminating demyelinising problem'. MS is thought to be a disease of the nervous system, but the earliest damage to nerve sheaths is caused by changes in the small blood vessels around the nerves. During the period 1963 to 1978 the number of hospital admissions for MS among men has remained the same but amongst women it has nearly doubled. This may well be a result of the pill since in experiments MS was found to be increased by the progestogen-only medroxy progesterone acetate (MPA).

Although the majority of western doctors in general practice prescribe the pill, very few have published detailed records and even fewer have looked directly at the blood vessel changes which so often match the symptoms. When I listed our patients alphabetically, irrespective of which pill they were on, nine out of ten women developed multiple complaints, and serious life-threatening symptoms and signs were recorded for *one woman in every ten*.

In 1982 Professor Victor Wynn of St Mary's Hospital, London, published the results of a study using the lowest dose combined pill available.[12] After three years only 8 per cent of the original 210 women were taking it. Out of thirty-nine women entering the third year, two developed deep venous thrombosis and one had a superficial thrombosis.

The problems just will not go away.

Summary

* The pill causes clots, abnormal blood cells, leg cramps, varicose veins, small distended surface veins, and changes to arteries and veins throughout the body

* Longer pill use causes more vessel changes

* Vessels of the womb at hysterectomy are still abnormal several years after stopping the pill in many women

* So-called microdose pills are still causing thrombosis

(iii) Changes in the Brain: The Pill Makes You Blue

Common Belief: *The pill can be used to treat premenstrual tension.*

Fact: *Mood changes are the main reason most women stop the pill within three years.*

It has been known throughout history that women are likely to become moody and unpredictable at certain times each month. So close is the time-worn association of strange behaviour with monthly cycles that it has become part of our language. The word lunatic is derived from the Latin word for moon. It is this very fact that most women notice some mood changes each month that has led to the dismissal of the real, intense and sometimes dangerous mental changes caused by the contraceptive pill.

In the sixties, women in our pill trial who complained of depression, disinterest in sex, irritability and aggression, were dismissed as neurotic. I was determined to prove that their mood changes were real, affected by hormones and therefore measurable. I did this to my own satisfaction by the mid-sixties[1,2] but twenty years later this work has been mostly ignored.

Depression can be a fatal side-effect of the pill. After six years of observing effects on our volunteer women we were able to predict the present rise in cases of battered children, and of suicides. A decade later research workers were reporting dramatic rises in self-poisoning and self-injury with the greatest increases occurring in females aged between fifteen and thirty. (The Oxford/FPA study[3] found pill users were four times more likely to be admitted to hospital for attempting suicide than those women who used the diaphragm.) The steepest increase was in the fifteen to nineteen age group — mostly single young women, classified as depressed in the researchers' tables. Girls in this group have been pressurised into taking the pill for its reliability and convenience.

Depression and loss of libido are most likely with progestogenic pills with a low dose of oestrogen. Women need oestrogen to keep them happy and a low dose oestrogen pill tends to make them more miserable. These pills may have protected women from some of the more frightening physical risks but they carry mental strains and these are tolerated by the medical profession as a lesser, preferable side-effect.

Our early pill research led to the discovery that in a normal cycle there is a dramatic rise in an enzyme (catalyst) called monoamine oxidase towards the end of the month and this is the time women feel unhappy or tense and irritable. Drugs which suppress monoamine oxidase (MAO) are therefore often given to patients in depressed states. We found that more than a quarter of women taking strongly progestogenic pills with a low dose of oestrogen became depressed, and two out of 136 women taking the first pill we tested were sufficiently depressed to attempt suicide. Most of them also complained of losing interest in sexual intercourse. These pills had especially high MAO levels.

There were other mood changes noted too, including some *increased* libidos — not entirely surprising as the pills are made from male hormones. One patient, a beauty therapist, complained of growing dark body hairs. Another pill, with male hormone-like actions and a slightly *higher* balance of oestrogen, had a peculiar effect on sex drive and mood. Mrs E, for example, went on a bus trip and had to suppress an overwhelming desire to hug and kiss the driver! This was quite out of character she told me.

Only a few women discontinued their tablets because of mood changes during the early cycles but over the whole trial 40 per cent of those withdrawing because of side-effects had at least one mood complaint. Mrs E's pill, which resembles some still being marketed, had particularly severe mood effects of aggression, violence and amnesia.

Mrs N was twenty-three. She had been happily taking a pill for two years when she was changed to the pill Mrs E was taking. Gradually over the next ten months she got more irritable. One day she exploded with anger at her husband and threw a frozen chicken at him. Luckily he was unhurt, but he had to tell her about the attack as she had lost her memory and couldn't remember what had happened. Another lady on the same pill threw a large biscuit tin at her husband. Although this pill did not depress it seemed particularly likely to cause violent mood swings.

Deaths through suicide or accidents are not often considered to be due to the pill and are therefore not reported. And until the evidence is widely accepted that the pill increases the risk of death through mental illness or violence they will continue to be overlooked.

Premenstrual Syndrome

Over the past fifty years scientific papers have been published establishing that women are more likely to have accidents or commit crimes before or during their periods. One reported how women airpilots were more likely to crash, another described how French women prisoners convicted of violent crimes had committed 85 per cent of their offences in the critical premenstrual phase.

In this country Dr Katharina Dalton has popularised the premenstrual syndrome.[4] She found the French study repeated here — women were more likely to commit crimes before a period. She took the matter further and found that children's illnesses can also depend on their mothers' cycles. Not only are women more likely to be off work, sick or admitted to hospital at period times, but their children are also more at risk of being taken to a doctor or admitted to hospital. Some mothers realised they had been unnecessarily violent with their children just before their periods when their feelings of tension were unbearable.

Premenstrual symptoms are part of a normal cycle and they can be distressing enough. But they last for only a few critical days and the majority of women learn to adapt to them in their own way. A few women are less sensitive and seem unaffected by their hormone changes but they are unusual. The pill changes this radically. Most oral contraceptives produce changes like those in the premenstrual phase. But instead of this critical time lasting just a few days, it can stretch over several weeks.

It is a mixed and complicated picture. Some women report that their PMT diminishes on the pill. With our first pill we found 26 per cent experienced less tension, 11 per cent said it was worse and 5 per cent felt no change. With regulated hormones there are not the sudden swings in enzymes and this has been claimed as a benefit. However, synthetic and naturally derived hormone preparations can mask premenstrual symptoms *for a short time*. What happens then is that each type of hormone or dose combination has particular symptoms which can intensify and remain throughout the cycle.

More Discoveries

While I was wondering how to prove that mood changes were real and not psychological, an important discovery was made in pharmacology with implications for psychiatry — and my own research. As is often the case in medicine, developments can come as spin-offs from unrelated research. In this case, a drug known to block the enzyme mono amine oxidase, was given to patients with tuberculosis.

A surprise result was that the patients who had been depressed suddenly felt much better.

There was great excitement aroused by the unexpected benefit and MAO inhibitor drugs became widely used in psychiatry to treat depression. Then there was the inevitable side-effect. Some of the patients got excruciating headaches and some even developed brain haemorrhages. These reactions were especially likely if they had also eaten cheese, chocolate or drunk alcohol.

This effect, however, helped advance our knowledge of the body's regulating mechanisms. Our circulation is continually changing in response to the environment. Blood vessels constrict if we are cold and dilate if we are hot, and if they over-react some of us have headaches or migraine. From research work over the past twenty years we know that the main chemicals responsible for this blood vessel and brain reactivity are called amines, which are made in our bodies from the proteins we eat. Cheese, especially the mouldy variety, is packed with tyr*amine*, chocolate has lots of phenylethyl*amine* and alcohol is high in hist*amine*. Migraine is induced in susceptible people if they eat too much of any of these. As the amine levels rise in their blood, their vessels tend to over-react and give them pain. MAO is one of the enzymes which helps to break down the proteins and amines in our bodies. If there are high levels of enzyme activity, the amine levels fall too drastically and cause depression. But when the enzyme's action was blocked by the new medicine, the amine levels sometimes rose too quickly causing spasm and haemorrhage. This is why the MAO-inhibitor drugs for depression carried warnings to patients to give cheese, chocolate and alcohol a wide berth.

A paper in the *Lancet*[5] at that time described how there were changes in MAO activity in the lining of the womb just before a woman's normal cyclic bleeding. As soon as I saw this paper I thought it gave a clue to the high depressive mood change with some contraceptive pills. By then I had realised that only some pills caused immediate depression and loss of libido and these were mostly progestogenic with the late secretory phase in the endometrium prolonged from two or three days to two or three weeks. I wondered whether the depression-inducing pills increased MAO activity more than others. With this question in my mind I rushed off to see Professor Merton Sandler who had been helping me investigate the pill headaches in the Department of Chemical Pathology at Queen Charlotte's Maternity Hospital. He was not impressed, but his pathologist colleague Dr John Pryse-Davies stepped in to help by promising to stain our endometrial samples to see whether the MAO activity was strong, weak or moderate.

I collected samples in the usual way and froze them immediately for their journey. The little bottles were put in a thermos and a special delivery boy took them on the back of his motorcycle to Queen Charlotte's. Apart from one day when the thermos exploded and we lost the specimens, we were to carry out his regular chore for two years until we had six groups of results.

They were even more conclusive than I had imagined. Besides MAO, two other enzymes — alkaline and acid phosphatases were also measured. At that time I did not know the significance of the other two enzymes but we now know that alkaline phosphatase is important for absorption in the gut and possibly connected with the development of food allergies.

All three were altered by steroid hormones.[2]

My suspicion that the very depressive pills might cause greater MAO changes in the endometrium was confirmed — sure enough, these pills produced high MAO activity for nearly the whole month.

This was very exciting, because once more it seemed obvious that what was happening in the lining of the womb was matching what was going on elsewhere in the body. One in four women became depressed with the higher dose progestogen pills but only if they also have a low dose of oestrogen. Of 214 women taking these big dose progestogen, low dose oestrogen compounds, 28 per cent complained of depressive mood changes compared with 6 per cent of the 301 women taking the oestrogen sequentials. The rate for the 702 women taking other pills was between 16 per cent and 20 per cent, but these weaker progestogenic pills caused more irregular bleeding. One high dose pill which gave a high MAO — due to the progestogen — did not depress women but it also contained a high dose of oestrogen and only 3 per cent were affected. The lower dose progestogen and low oestrogen pills now commonly used can now cause depression in about one in ten women.

It became clear to me that oestrogen increases amine production and prevents depression but too much progestogen causes depression, presumably by increasing amine break-down and lowering tissue levels. Tiredness and irritability were more likely with the weaker doses but these, of course, also cause more irregular bleeding, and increased pregnancy risk. What we were suggesting was not eagerly greeted. We sent our results to a clinical biochemical journal in the United States to have it returned, about a year later, with the comment that it was *ludicrously unscientific to suggest that a chemical change in the womb could be connected with brain changes.*

But when Dr Sandler saw how well our results had worked out he agreed to measure MAO biochemically, and in 1967 we were ready to publish the changes in the normal cycle. We had discovered that the rise in MAO activity was dramatic, ranging from below 1,000 to more than 20,000 units of activity. The high levels were only found in the late secretory specimens — meaning that women have to cope with as much as a twenty times change in enzyme activity just before a period.[6] MAO activity in the blood increases, then falls before the period begins. The latest research, twenty years after our discovery, makes the connection between brain and womb changes more likely.

Animals Too

Techniques now available show how different areas in the brain respond to hormone and amine stimuli. While the effect of the natural hormone progesterone has not yet been shown to alter brain MAO in women, particular areas are being mapped out in animals' brains according to their reactions to hormone and amine stimuli.

In the sixties Dr Richard Michael, working at the Institute of Psychiatry, gave progesterone to female monkeys and found they were less interested in the males who, incidentally, became less interested in them. He discovered that vaginal secretions contain copulins which are made by normal vaginal bacteria. Progesterone changed the vaginal cells, just as it alters cells in the womb, and the bacteria produced less copulin. Dr Michael also discovered that the same process happens in women taking the pill. [7]

In women it is known that oestrogens are converted into highly active 'catechol' oestrogens which control amine metabolism in the sensitive areas of the brain and in target organs like the uterus and ovaries. It is not ludicrous to suggest that womb changes might give a more direct indication of changes in the brain than measurements of blood levels.

The sequential pills, oestrogen only for the first eleven or fifteen days, had low MAO throughout the cycle. Adding a progestogen for the last ten or fifteen days did not increase the MAO activity and few women became depressed taking these pills. One company, manufacturing sequentials, wanted enough copies of our paper, published by the *BMJ* [2] in 1968, to circulate every GP in Australia. The *BMJ* refused to issue so many reprints. Just as well, as later it was discovered that giving oestrogen alone had greatly increased the incidence of endometrial cancer in the USA.

Mood changes are not only caused by progesterone-oestrogen mixtures. Although oestrogen is commonly used to treat depression, either oestrogen or progesterone given alone can cause many serious metabolic upsets, including dramatically raising levels of blood copper in susceptible women — those who have a tendency to schizophrenia.

Mrs MK had been taking oestrogens for years. She was given 'natural' mare's oestrogens when she felt ill after a hysterectomy and removal of her ovaries in her late thirties. When she tried to do without the hormones she became breathless, so she restarted the oestrogens and felt well again.

She looked young for her age, her hair and skin were lovely, she dressed well and she was happily looking after her children. But gradually Mrs MK became more and more anxious, restless and upset. She became worried about the children, felt trapped in her beautiful home and felt life had no future for her.

By now she was seeing a psychiatrist who was giving her anti-depressants. Neither she nor the psychiatrist believed that her condition was affected by taking oestrogens; they both thought her problems were mental. She had been told that oestrogens were given to treat menopausal depression and she was sure her symptoms were due to lack of oestrogens if she didn't take them. The anti-depressants made her much worse however. She became violent, and sadly, her second suicide attempt ended with her death.

For some women, no amount of conjuring could come up with a symptom-free pill. This is what happened when we tried to get it right for three women.

Mrs NL took a low dose progestogen, high dose oestrogen pill (ethynodiol diacetate 0.1mg + mestranol 0.1mg) for nineteen months. She asked to change to something else because of heavy irregular bleeding with cramps and numbness in her feet. Her endometrial biopsy showed lots of dilated sinusoids.

She changed to the 1mg dose of the same pill. Her leg and feet symptoms disappeared and her periods became very scanty. This time she wanted to stop after only three months because she had lost interest in sex. Although this pill was strongly progestogenic the effect of the high dose of oestrogen made some women have vein symptoms and two out of thirty women developed thrombophlebitis.

Mrs NL then tried a sequential pill with the same high dose of oestrogen for twenty-one days and a progestogen (chloramadinone 2mg) added for ten days. She still complained of depression and loss of libido and changed once more to the 0.25mg dose of ethynodiol diacetate plus mestranol. She took it for fourteen months but had irregular bleeding for eleven of these cycles.

Mrs ID started on the same low progestogen, high oestrogen pill but after twenty-seven months bled continuously for thirty-five days. She changed to the 0.25mg dose but bled for fifteen days after seven cycles and she complained of dizziness. Her next pill was the 0.5mg dose which she took for thirteen months before stopping it because of headaches, dizziness, severe cramps in her right leg and putting on 14lb in weight.

Of the twenty other patients trying this particular pill, one collapsed with severe chest pain, one was admitted to hospital for an acute anxiety state and another for abdominal pains.

Mrs VO took three different doses of norgestrel with low dose of oestrogen. She was thirty-seven and had ten children with no miscarriages.

She had suffered premenstrual tension, depression and headaches before her periods and occasional leg cramps. She started with 0.1mg of norgestrel and after nine cycles she had two irregular bleeding cycles, more leg cramps than usual and her varicose veins had burst on two occasions.

She then took the 0.25mg dose for twelve months and gained 9lb in weight. She was changed to the 0.5mg dose because the lower dose had been discontinued for causing too much breakthrough bleeding. Twelve months later she stopped the pill altogether as she had developed swollen fingers and ankles, was fainting and had feelings of tightness in her chest.

We found repeatedly that varying either the dose of progestogen or oestrogen changed the women's symptoms from breakthrough bleeding to vein effects, to arterial effects like headache and high blood pressure, to weight gain, to depression. So-called 'neurotic' symptoms like tiredness, anxiety and irritability were most marked with the mid range pills which had a higher balance of oestrogen. All pills were producing numerous side-effects sooner or later. The results of our London Trials, it seemed to me, were that high doses caused a wide range of side-effects while low doses caused as many pregnancies as mechanical methods of contraception.

Violence to Children

Since 1961 the numbers of children taken into care increased every year up to 1980. Violence to babies has become so common in the past twenty years that it is a well-known reason for children being admitted to hospital.

Women who feel tired and depressed are less likely to have patience with their babies when they cry. Violence is known to be connected with alcoholism, post-partum depression, lead pollution, split families, lack of caring relatives and many other social reasons but it is a pity that violence to children has not been investigated thoroughly in the major pill studies. Women in our trial told us that they felt murderous towards their children when they were taking the pill, but immediately felt better when they stopped taking it. Some women also became aggressive to their husbands. The original very high doses of pills used at first in America mimicked pregnancy but lower dose pills simulate immediately after childbirth when thrombosis, depression, irrational violent behaviour are most likely when hormone levels have fallen.

Jacqueline was twenty-five when she came to consult me. She had been taking 'lots of different pills on and off' since she was sixteen. She couldn't remember all their names but they were mostly 'low dose' pills.

When she was nineteen, she had been walking along the road with her boyfriend, and suddenly burst into tears for no apparent reason. She didn't know why she felt so miserable. She went to her general practitioner who gave her tranquillisers. A few months later in December she took an overdose. The following August she was admitted to hospital after a second attempt on her life which was nearly successful. By this time Jacqueline was having frequent migraine attacks. She felt sick and dizzy and had a bad taste in her mouth. The skin on her brow had become pigmented. She finally stopped the pill when she was twenty-two. The pigment disappeared and the migraine attacks improved.

She used a copper intrauterine device for a year but it had to be taken out because of heavy, irregular bleeding. When I saw her for the first time, she had become allergic to many foods and chemicals. She had continuous headaches and felt faint when she cooked with gas.

She had had several boyfriends and was now engaged to be married. When her fiancé returned from Canada and saw how ill she was, he broke off the engagement. Close personal relationships had become very difficult. This is one of the penalties for ex-pill takers who have not recovered their health.

Depression after childbirth can lead a mother to violence. After pregnancy a woman's hormone levels suddenly fall, giving a steroid withdrawal effect on the brain. But there is another important cause of post-partum depression or psychosis. A pregnant and lactating woman needs extra zinc for her growing child. Zinc is concentrated in the placenta and lost at child-birth. Animals replace their zinc by eating their placentae. If a woman has been taking the pill she is more likely to be zinc deficient at the start of her pregnancy. As zinc supplements are not usually taken by most pregnant mothers, this means that post-partum zinc deficiency, severe enough to induce depression, will have become more common among mothers. The children themselves are also more likely to have zinc deficiency and mineral imbalance which can cause anti-social behaviour and I shall discuss this in greater depth in Chapter 8.

Divorce

A number of women gave break-up of their marriage as a reason for ceasing to come to our pill clinic in the sixties. This may not have had much impact on us then but in looking back it can be seen as the start of a divorce epidemic which by 1983 had affected nearly one third of all marriages. The 1974 study of the Royal College of General Practitioners found that divorce was twice as common among pill users.

Suicide

In the 1930s there were three men attempting suicide for every one woman (if this may be ascribed to the effects of the

Depression, it should be remembered that these were bad times for women too.) By 1980, the sex ratios had been reversed. It is now three women for each man.

Since the late sixties there had been a dramatic increase in suicide attempts by women, and especially in the fifteen to nineteen age group. During 1968 one poisoning treatment centre in Edinburgh[8] admitted 307 girls, six years later they were dealing with 560 a year.

Since 1962 suicide attempts have increased by 6 per cent for men but by 13 per cent for women. The men tend to be criminals, alcoholics or drug addicts but the sexes have one thing in common — both are likely to have suffered a recent break-up of a close relationship prior to their attempt.

This dramatic increase in suicide attempts by young women has happened in most western countries since the pill was introduced.[9] Five years before the pill, suicide attempts in the USA were estimated at 15 per 100,000 of the population a year. By 1977, nearly one in a hundred young women in the fifteen to twenty-four age group[10] was trying to kill herself every year. This was a few years after the higher oestrogen pills had been discontinued.

I have seen several young women who have made repeated attempts on their lives when they were taking the pill. For many women, the amount of oestrogen in a low dose pill is just not enough to keep them happy, especially as their own oestrogen production is blocked by the pill.

Accidental Deaths

Accidents and violence are the number one cause of death among fifteen to twenty-four year olds. Although it is a common belief that a women is more likely to be killed in a traffic accident than die from taking the pill, in fact data from controlled trials show that women taking the pill have an increased risk of accidents compared with other women.

In 1980 the large American Walnut Creek contraceptive

study reported a higher risk of accidental poisonings, suicide and murder among pill users[11] while the Royal College of General Practitioners mortality data published in 1981 showed pill takers had twice the number of accidental deaths.[12] In England and Wales accidental poisonings and undetermined deaths increased eleven fold among males aged fifteen to nineteen but twenty-two times among young women since 1960.[13] The 1984 RCGP report showed significant increases in attempted suicides (283 amongst pill takers, to 106 amongst controls). Events related to pregnancy and post-partum were omitted.

Schizophrenia

The pill hormones can raise copper levels in most women, but schizophrenics can have exceptionally high copper levels[14]. Very high copper levels have been found in women in pre-eclampsia post-partum depression, and psychosis. Schizophrenic psychosis can be precipitated by steriod withdrawal, such as stopping the pill.

At the request of the Schizophrenia Association of Great Britain I reviewed how biochemical and immune changes caused by the pill and smoking could precipitate mental illness in susceptible people.[15] In theory fluctuations in the same chemicals can decide whether a person becomes depressed, gets migraine attacks or suffers from schizophrenia.

Summary

* With many of the pills premenstrual tension is increased from a few days each month to three weeks

* Higher progestogen pills with low oestrogen bring about loss of libido in 1 in 4 women

59

* Pills causing high MAO activity combined with a low dose of oestrogen cause most depression

* Changes in alkaline and acid phosphatases (secretory enzymes) increase risk of reactions to food

* High copper with low zinc levels leads to increased risk of schizophrenia and mental illness

* Controversy has arisen because large doses of pill steroids may temporarily suppress symptoms

3 Swings and Roundabouts: Upsets in Metabolism

Common belief: *By switching doses of oestrogen and progestogen you can lose the metabolic side-effects.*

Fact: *Oestrogens and progestogens have different effects on fats, proteins and carbohydrates so it hasn't been possible to find a pill which is free from unwanted side-effects.*

Gall Bladder Disease

Alison was a young mother of two children. She was thirty years old and she looked healthy, bright and cheerful. She was a statistician and I asked her to help me when I was preparing the results of the London Trials for the *BMJ* in 1965. She calculated that the differences in numbers of women having headaches, thrombosis or depression were highly significant with different pills. This means that the symptoms had not just happened by chance but were more likely than not caused by the different doses of hormones.

Our daughters were in the same class at nursery school so we visited each other for tea. One summer day I brought Alison a large strawberry cream cake. She looked at it longingly and said 'That looks lovely but I can't eat fatty foods. I'm going to have my gall bladder taken out in a week or two.' I commiserated with her but then suddenly thought to ask her if she was on the pill. Alison said she was. On my advice she stopped the pill at once. The surgeon was amazed that the gall stones he had seen on Alison's X-rays disappeared before he could operate. Nearly twenty years later Alison still has her gall bladder and she has no difficulty in eating fatty food after stopping the pill.

I first noticed that some of the pill research volunteers were developing gall bladder disease in the early sixties and notified the Committee on Safety of Drugs. These were the first notifications they had but soon other cases were reported in Britain. Gall bladder disease was no longer just for the 'fair, fat, fertile and forty' but was becoming more common in younger women than ever before. Gall bladder disease increases with the pill because oestrogens raise cholesterol levels while progestogens delay emptying — both making cholesterol gall stones more likely.

Weight Gain or Anorexia

One of the best known pill side-effects is weight gain. Again, before the days of the pill, obesity was linked to the menopause and known as 'middle-aged spread'. Oddly enough, weight gain does not depend just on the doses of hormones in a pill but depends as much on the exact hormone balance of each pill. With one pill, which had a medium dose of progestogen and a low dose of oestrogen, half of the women gained ten pounds in their first year. Mrs GD for example, had headaches during her first cycle. Her legs became sore and she felt more tired each day. By ten months she had put on 21lb. She stopped taking the pill and her weight reverted to normal within a few months.

While I did not review weight gain for a separate paper for a medical journal, I found that it was the pills which caused the biggest vascular and mood effects, which also had the greatest effect on weight gain. In spite of each pill having particular biochemical actions, not all women are affected equally. Some gain weight rapidly, others only gain weight very slowly and they may not connect their obesity with taking the pill or hormone replacement therapy. Some lose their appetites. They are unable to eat, get thinner and become anorexic. When forced to eat they may get fatter and fatter as the normal controlling mechanisms have been disrupted. But the pill works by blocking the normal controlling mechanisms in the brain, the hypothalamus and pituitary gland.

Unfortunately the pill not only interferes with the normal control of sexual function but it can also interfere with the hormones which regulate stress, growth, thyroid activity, and the breakdown and metabolism of our food — carbohydrates, proteins, fats, trace minerals, vitamins and our salt and water balance.

When steroid hormones like the pill are taken into the body, they alter the production of other steroid hormones made in the adrenal glands. (See Appendix I for a more detailed review.) Dr Kitty Little has described how pill steroids cause abnormalities in bones, blood cells, blood vessels and stress coping mechanisms. In animal experiments, she discovered that young immature animals had the greatest changes and her work has made her extremely concerned about the risk of long-term osteoporosis (thinning of bone tissue), joint and back problems in young girls given the pill at puberty — a time when their bodies often have difficulty adjusting to adult hormone patterns anyway. As early as 1968 Dr Little predicted an increase in premature senile symptoms among pill users and particularly an increase in stress fractures among young women taking it. Ballet teachers in London have complained that their pupils are now having many more unexpected fractures and young women athletes are also being affected.

Diabetes and Heart Disease

Professor Victor Wynn and his team at St Mary's Hospital, Paddington have shown how the pill can cause diabetes. Progesterone and progestogens (in minute doses) can raise the blood sugar and cause a resistance to insulin, as do the male hormones and anabolic steroids used by some athletes.

Oestrogens are especially likely to raise the production of

blood fats like cholesterol but progestogens, with male hormone-like actions, lower a special fraction of cholesterol. Low levels of this HLD_2 fraction have been associated with increasing the risk of arterial disease. This is thought to be a contributory factor to why women on the pill have a greater risk of heart disease.

Body Chemistry

Protein metabolism can be switched around by the pill and progestogens tend to slow the activity of the enzymes in the liver which clean our blood. Proteins are broken down by abnormal pathways and abnormal chemicals appear in the urine. A shortage of zinc and vitamin B_6 can develop causing more upsets to carbohydrate metabolism and cellular metabolism in general.

Although we found that oestrogens decreased and progestogens increased MAO activity, another enzyme which breaks down proteins, COMT, was either too high or too low in the blood of women taking the same pill. Both of

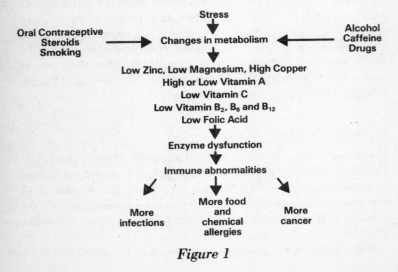

Figure 1

these enzymes need the trace element copper but the pill increases copper levels too much, especially in susceptible women.

The pill can cause too low zinc and too high copper which, in turn, may disrupt gut and liver function leading to food reactions and even anorexia or bulimia. The pill can also upset iron, magnesium, manganese, iodine and chromium levels and these can be diagnosed by mineral analysis.

To illustrate how steroid hormones can affect trace mineral metal levels in the body, a patient taking so-called natural oestrogens and a progestogen for over ten years, had a detailed mineral analysis of blood, hair and sweat. There were very severe zinc, magnesium and manganese deficiencies, with very high copper. She was given mineral and vitamin supplements while the oestrogens were gradually stopped, avoiding the otherwise inevitable withdrawal side-effects. Weindling and Henry reviewed laboratory tests altered by the pill,[1] and the vitamin changes will be discussed in more detail in Chapter 8 and Appendix I.

The Latest Pills — too much or too little testosterone?

When Professor Wynn reported that even a low dose of l-norgestrel was still causing metabolic changes interest swung to the weaker desogestrel which has a strong progesterone-like action but almost no androgen or anti-oestrogen effect. The results on trials of Marvelon — 150 micrograms desogestrel and 30 micrograms ethinyl oestradiol — were reported in 1983 at a workshop on oral contraception.[2] It was found to have a similar incidence of side-effects and breakthrough bleeding as a low dose triphasic containing l-norgestrel and ethinyl oestradiol. Only one pregnancy occurred among 427 women. The effects on metabolism were those of the accompanying oestrogen — the blood fats were raised as well as the plasma proteins. Levels of testosterone were very low.

Most oral contraceptives lower the levels of free testosterone. Normally women have a peak interest in initiating sexual activity in the middle of their cycles at ovulation and most oral contraceptives take away this peak effect so that there is a significant reduction in sexual intercourse. Pills with no androgen (male hormones) activity used to treat acne and hairiness and polycystic ovary disease, result in very low testosterone levels. A Swedish professor commented 'We have a hard time keeping our women on some of the various experimental models of treatment.' It seemed that these women preferred to be hairy, keep their libido and not take drugs! He also noted that the Swedish Regulatory Board, heavily dominated by very active women, is very sceptical of any combination that decreases testosterone levels. Hirsutism is claimed to be very common among pill users, and some Swedish investigators think that the powerful androgenic progestogens like norgestrel can cause hairiness by displacing binding sites and releasing endogenous testosterone.

During the workshop concern was expressed over the prolonged action of a progestogen (which is in a pill widely recommended for adolescent girls' acne, but not boys who have more acne) made it difficult to get patients to menstruate unless they were given extra oestrogen. (In fact acne often responds dramatically to zinc supplementation and a low allergy diet.) The speaker also felt there was a need for a suitable pill for hirsute women particularly since the relatively non-androgenic pills had been removed from the market for causing breast lumps in beagle dogs.

Twenty-five years on and the oral contraceptive scene is still going round in circles. Even taking the same pill, the levels of some critical controlling enzymes go too high or too low. It is a game of swings and roundabouts. Very few people realise that because of individual variations of the enzymes in the gut wall and liver, blood levels of pill progestogens can vary up to *ten times*.[3] Self medication with large doses of the usually beneficial vitamin C has the effect of upgrading a pill from a low to a high dose of oestrogen.

Summary

* The pill interferes with:
  the normal coordination between the brain and the pituitary gland
  normal control of sexual function
  stress coping mechanisms
  growth hormones
  thyroid activity
  the breakdown, absorption and metabolism of carbo-hydrates, fats and proteins
  liver function
  trace mineral balance
  salt and water control
  bone, blood cell and blood vessel development
  immune function including prostaglandin and antibody formation

* All of this can lead to more infections, more food and chemical allergy weight problems such as anorexia or obesity, osteoporosis and cancer.

4   Even Worse than Smoking

Common belief: *If women on the pill give up smoking they run fewer risks of vascular and other diseases.*

Fact: *The pill by itself causes more vascular disease and cancer than smoking alone does.*

By the early 1970s we had tried every possible pill combination and it was clear to me that however the two pill hormones were altered or manipulated they still provoked too much illness. The pill was a convenience rather than a medical necessity and I thought women would eventually turn to other methods.

By this time the world's medical literature had reported nearly every known medical illness as a possible or definite side-effect of the pill and it could no longer be claimed as the ideal form of contraceptive. A more comprehensive approach was tried by the medical profession rather than the blanket pill prescription. The slogan was 'Whichever method suits each woman best'. In practice that usually means try the pill first, then the coil or IUD, followed by cap or sheath, or pessaries, or sterilisation.

I turned my attention from testing pills for the Family Planning Association and followed up a suggestion made to me by Dr Raymond Greene, the eminent endocrinologist, that I study migraine. He pointed me to the Migraine Trust which had been set up in 1965, at a time when an increasing number of younger women were reporting migraine. The Trust had started the Princess Margaret Migraine Clinic in London for on the spot treatment of emergency headaches suffered by office workers. A doctor was always on duty to treat acute cases, and also to take referrals from GPs.

Research was carried out in collaboration with neighbouring hospitals.

I was invited to work some locum sessions at the clinic by its director Dr Marcia Wilkinson. I also started regular clinics at the Royal Surrey County Hospital in Guildford, as an assistant to the neurologist Dr Desmond Carrol. Later I joined the research team of Dr Frank Clifford Rose in the Neurology Department at Charing Cross Hospital which now also houses the Princess Margaret Migraine Clinic. At all three clinics I found I saw far more women, and most of the younger ones were on the pill but most of the men were smokers.

Smoking

Soon, patterns of class emerged in the smoking habits of patients attending the clinics at Charing Cross and Guildford. Both had some very heavily smoking men but there were fewer female smokers in Guildford, a well-off country district, than around the Charing Cross, which is in a working-class area of London. In the previous twenty years what we had learned about smoking causing cancer and vascular disease had seen a drop in the number of people smoking among the higher social classes to 25 per cent of men and women. But in the lowest social class (V) 61 per cent of men and 42 per cent of women still smoked.

I had become more interested in smoking because the serious vascular complications of the pill were the same as those caused by smoking, which suggested to me that there might be some similar underlying mechanism. A side-effect of both is headache but I found that while the *average* man or woman smoker went to the hospital migraine clinics after smoking twenty cigarettes a day for twenty-five years, the average contraceptive pill user was coming after three to four years of pill use.

Heart Attacks

In 1974 a German doctor calculated that heart attacks were unusual in smokers until they had smoked more than 200,000 cigarettes (at least twenty cigarettes per day for twenty-five years) and the heaviest smokers coming to our clinics had reached this total. The young women pill-taking smokers who had averaged 59,130 cigarettes — eighteen a day for nine years — had been on the pill for three years. Most of the premature vascular deaths happen to women who have taken the pill for between one and six years — clearly a much shorter fuse than for smoking.

Dr Glynn Volans, a young registrar at the Princess Margaret Clinic, had noticed that many migraine patients disliked tobacco smoke, especially during their attacks. As he already knew that smokers have raised levels of carboxy haemoglobin (COHb) — due to carbon monoxide from cigarette smoke replacing oxygen in red blood cells — and as he also knew that COHb could cause vasodilation and headaches, Volans arranged to measure COHb levels in migraine patients. Surprisingly, in his 1976 paper with Castledon, he concluded that smoking was unlikely to be a factor in causing migraine as smokers with headaches did not have higher levels of COHb than headache-free smokers.[1] They had also expected to find more smokers among migraine patients than in the general population but in fact they found fewer and among women referred to the clinic for a second opinion, there were four times fewer smokers than expected. I also noticed this but found emergency patients were more likely to be smokers.

Migraine

When I charted patients' headaches over three months I came up with some highly significant statistics. For example, thirty pill users totalled 424 days with migraine compared with 128 days for the same number of non-users. Smokers

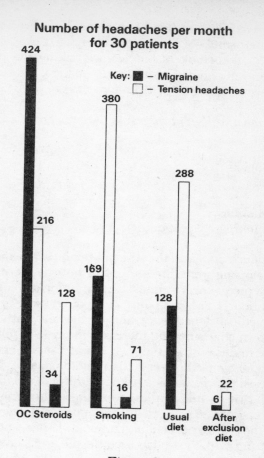

Number of headaches per month for 30 patients

Key: ■ – Migraine
□ – Tension headaches

Figure 2

had 169 days with migraine but 380 days with 'tension' headaches. While pill users suffered the most migraine, smokers had most tension headaches. Many of the regular ergotamine users were addicted to the drug and would immediately have migraine attacks if they forgot to take it every morning.

When we grouped together both emergency and referred

patients according to these habits we discovered that men and women smokers were more likely to make emergency visits than non-smokers but women taking the pill made even more emergency visits than smokers. Most of these women were taking so-called micro-dosage pills.

Percentage of different migraine patients given acute treatment

	Male	Female
Non-smokers	15	10
Smokers	35	33
Pill	—	49
Pill & smoking	—	57
Pill & smoking & ergotamine	—	78

The evidence indicates that the pill can be worse than smoking for causing migraine and using both is more likely to cause frequent, severe attacks. Ergotamine use complicates the situation.[2,3] This is a point which often escapes attention in the medical debate surrounding the pill. Although it is well-known that smoking increases the risk of pill-induced vascular disease[4] of all types, it is not usually emphasised that the pill by itself is worse than smoking alone. Yet it was this pattern which emerged from reports of deaths during the two big British pill studies.[5,6] Of the eighty-one vascular deaths recorded, 6 per cent of the women had never smoked or used the pill, 10 per cent had smoked, 19 per cent had used the pill, and 65 per cent had used the pill and smoked. This, of course, was presented to the public as proof that if you avoid smoking, the pill is safe.

Two studies, the Oxford/FPA and Walnut Creek, also found significantly increased risks of cervical cancer in young women smokers but their data showed that pill takers had a much greater risk of cervical cancer than smokers.[7]

Incidence of cervical cancer

		Pill	Non Pill	Smoking	Non Smoking
1978 Oxford/FPA	All	30†	9*	21	18
1981 Walnut Creek	Under 40	37	1	14	18

*Seven were IUD users and two were diaphragm users.
†All six cases of invasive cancers were in pill users.

Tranquillisers

It is interesting that smokers are especially prone to tension headaches, when most of them say they smoke to relieve tension. It is not such a paradox, as the relief gained by smoking often has a rebound effect. Smokers take more tranquillisers than non-smokers, something I discovered at the clinics. I found that nearly one in five of all smokers were taking regular Valium at their first visit but less than half as many ex-smokers were still taking this drug. When women were enrolled in the Walnut Creek study it was found that those who were taking or who had taken the pill were more likely to be taking tranquillisers. There has been an enormous rise in the prescribing of anti-depressants and tranquillisers to young women since smoking and the pill became commonplace. Many of these prescriptions are given to mask symptoms and they simply help people to carry on smoking and taking the pill. There are now one in five women taking tranquillisers compared to one in ten men. How many of the women I wonder who started on them when they were taking the pill have since found themselves addicted to them even after they have switched to another method of contraception?

Food

Dr Edda Hanington, who was running a migraine clinic at the Middlesex Hospital, London, had asked her patients which foods they thought gave them migraine. Some were unaware of a connection with their diet and their headaches but many others had noticed if they ate cheese, chocolate or oranges or drank alcohol — especially red wine — they often had a severe attack a few hours later.[8] Dr Hanington's women patients also said these foods were more likely to upset them at period times or if they took the pill.

Following up this work, I asked my patients to avoid eating these migraine-precipitating foods and stop taking the pill, stop smoking and avoid taking any daily medicine. Each group of patients had a ten-fold reduction in the number of their migraine attacks. Many had no more headaches, although some had suffered from regular migraine for most of their lives. Nearly all patients improved enormously. Half of the smokers and a third of the pill takers had no more headaches or migraine attacks.

One spectacular success was of a woman of forty-six, sent along by her GP because she had suffered from migraine for twenty-two years and had been smoking since she was sixteen. For thirty years she had smoked between fifteen and twenty cigarettes a day and for the last three years before coming to the clinic had had daily headaches. This patient had taken numerous medicines for her condition which had been prescribed by hospital doctors. My advice was to quit smoking and avoid certain foods. She left coffee, chocolate and cream out of her diet and four years later she was completely migraine-free. Her interest in life revived.

Most women lose their side-effects as soon as they stop the pill but some patients still suffered migraine even after stopping and leaving out the rogue foods. They recovered, however, after following a full allergy elimination diet, the results of which generated enormous interest after I published them in the *Lancet* in 1978.[9] The important discovery was that it was what people are doing in their day-to-day lives, what they are eating, breathing and drinking that often decides their state of health. Hans Selye, in his many papers and books about the general adaptation syndrome, has described how individuals can cope with mental or physical stress for long periods before their coping mechanisms break down and they become ill. The adaptation period for smoking seems to be twenty to twenty-five years but only a few years for oral contraceptive steroids. This is strong evidence that the pill is more harmful to health than smoking.

Dr Kitty Little has noted that progestogenic steroids, given experimentally with cortisol to represent the effect of day-to-day stress, drastically changed the developing cells of the bone marrow which then produced abnormal blood cells and masses of sticky platelets. Sticky platelets are abnormally sensitive to rises in blood amines from food and drink and more likely to clot together, causing migraine or thrombotic episodes. In 1982 Dr Hanington[10] and her colleagues published results showing that patients whose migraine began for the first time when they started low dose pills had significantly more sticky platelets than other women. Four to six months after stopping the pill there was a marked improvement in symptoms and the platelets were less likely to clot when exposed to amines, like those in cheese, in the laboratory.

By now I knew that platelets, red cells and white blood cells can also change when we eat foods if we are allergic to them.

Summary

* The pill is more harmful than smoking. Users experience:

    more frequent and severe migraine attacks

premature deaths from vascular disease after only a few
    years of use
more emergency hospital visits
earlier incidence of cervical cancer
more invasive cervical cancer

both increase tranquilliser use

5 *Allergy, and How to Recover from the Pill*

> Common belief: *The effect of the pill on women's immune systems 'is unlikely to be of clinical importance', RCGP study 1974.*

> Fact: *Allergic and immune diseases have increased to epidemic proportions among women pill takers.*

Although there is now common agreement among doctors that women with migraine should not take the pill, many do not seem to realise that the pill is a major contributor to our present food allergy epidemic.

Behind the dramatic press stories of women who are 'allergic to the twentieth century' lies a disturbing trend. Women generally it seems have become more sensitive to chemicals, food and pollution.

Masking

At the heart of the pill controversy is the slowness of the medical profession to accept that not everyone is alike. The most sensitive of us react to medicines, drugs and hormones more quickly and intensely than the insensitive. Most of us react to some foods and chemicals but both we and our doctors are unaware of these reactions.

The difficulty in diagnosis is due to 'masking'. When we first take a food or other substance that upsets us we may dislike the taste or get a headache. However, if we go on taking it frequently our body adapts and we no longer have any warning symptoms although we may generally feel less well than we should. The length of this period of adaptation, or masking, is different for different substances. For example, we have just seen how the average smoker becomes obviously ill after an average of twenty-five years, but the average woman taking the pill becomes ill within two or three years. At this point, for most people, the body's regulatory mechanisms have become upset or maladapted giving continuous symptoms and more and more common foods and chemicals also begin to precipitate symptoms.

The diagnosis of these allergies can only be made, to the satisfaction of both patient and physician, when the patient stops taking the harmful substances, avoids eating common foods and avoids common chemicals like gas or traffic fumes. This can usually be done at home and only a few severe cases need to be admitted to a special environmental control unit so that they can fast in a room free from chemical contamination.

A further problem is that just as smoking or alcohol cause addiction and giving them up causes withdrawal symptoms, so common foods such as wheat, milk, sugar, tea and coffee can also be highly addictive and stopping them may cause surprisingly severe withdrawal symptoms.

The pill sometimes causes psychological dependence of a sort — with some women defensively justifying their need to continue taking hormones in spite of their obvious side-effects. Once they have given it up this feeling usually disappears and they become much more positive about using other methods of birth control or dealing with their menstrual or menopausal problems by more natural means, such as a healthy diet and exercise.

It took me about ten years to realise that immune changes played a key role in causing pill side-effects. Although headaches, vein and mood changes, irregular bleeding and weight changes depend on hormone doses and balance, they also depend on an individual's susceptibility. Women with an allergic family background usually get severe side-effects straightaway with whichever pill they are given. Other women may have a headache 24 hours after the first pill and not again until three or four years later when they may have daily headaches. By that time their coping mechanisms have become exhausted.

The key findings of our early pill trials were not just how side-effects vary with dose and type of pill, but how strikingly different individuals' susceptibilities to side-effects are. Doctors who want to give women injections of long-acting pill steroids of any variety, whose effects last three months, seem to be either unaware of this fact or taking a calculated risk.

It is an indisputable fact, however, that hormones have a profound effect on our immune system. Women are more reactive than men and pregnant women are even more sensitive. I always knew I was pregnant when I couldn't stand the taste of coffee! This is a protective mechanism — as little as one glass of wine a day in pregnancy is heavy drinking as far as the baby is concerned. So women's awareness of harmful substances is important.

What is Allergy?

Everyone thinks they know what allergy is — although doctors and scientists are busy arguing about exact definitions and disputing whether headaches are due to biochemical changes or immunological changes. A scientific experiment depends on isolating and investigating one particular aspect of the body's mechanisms, but, in a living body, changes in cells, chemicals and immune proteins all happen together or in sequence so that one change can trigger off more changes.

Our bodies are made up of millions of single cells. An amoeba is a tiny creature which has only one cell. When it meets even smaller viruses or bacteria, the amoeba engulfs them and secretes chemicals to digest them. We have developed special cells with these actions as part of our immune defence system. White cells in our blood attack invading bacteria and they secrete immune proteins (antibodies) to kill the invaders (antigens). If we produce too many antibodies and there are too many antigens, they all stick together in a lattice called an immune complex. This gives off a complement which makes platelets clot. The platelets secrete chemicals which dilate or constrict blood vessels, damage their walls and make even more platelets clot, causing headaches or thrombosis. But if we have too few antibodies, we are more vulnerable to tissue damage.

When a woman has sexual intercourse, the sperm are foreign to her body like invading bacteria but she does not usually destroy them. Her body does not reject the foreign protein of the father in the fertilised egg. As the baby grows in her womb, her oestrogen levels rise and stop the white cells attacking. Some women do reject the foetus and this can be a cause of habitual abortion. Reaction to the father's tissue may also be a reason for early pregnancy sickness. Oestrogens can increase antibody levels[1] and this means that pregnant women are more likely to have allergic reactions to food in the first three months. Progesterone has the opposite effect and lowers antibody formation.[2] The high levels of both steroid hormones during the last six months of pregnancy tend to suppress allergic reactions and give a feeling of well-being but a pregnant woman is more susceptible to infections and if she has a tumour it can grow more rapidly.

When the levels of hormones suddenly fall after the child is born, the mother may become more allergic once more. She may get thrombosis or post-partum depression. In so-called auto-immune conditions where the body reacts to its own tissues, diseases like multiple sclerosis (MS) are likely to flare-up. It is precisely at this critical time that long acting injections of progestogen-only contraceptives are being given. Experimentally, oestrogens suppress MS in animals but progestogens intensify and prolong the disease.[3] Progestogens are also more likely to intensify depression besides interfering with immune function.

Traditional medicine accepts that hay fever, asthma and skin rashes are caused by allergic reactions. Many individuals with these complaints have up to six times higher than usual amounts of an antibody called immunoglobulin E — IgE for short — in their blood. These patients are called atopic. Only a few women react to contraceptive pills in an acceptedly allergic way. One of our volunteers got asthma with a low dose pill but not with a high dose one. A few developed skin rashes and ear, nose and throat surgeons reported women taking the pill often had rhinitis and hay fever. I began to suspect that allergy might be involved in the development of all common pill side-effects because of one unusual migraine patient.

Mrs YG was an attractive, intelligent thirty-year-old, who had been attending Guildford migraine clinic for several years. When I first met her in 1972, she told me she had always had severe reactions to hormone changes. She had always had headaches and usually migraine with her periods. As a child she had recurrent infections but no one else in the family had migraine and her parents did not smoke. When she was twenty-five she was prescribed an oral contraceptive pill to see if it would help her menstrual migraine. The result was devastating. After taking the second tablet she collapsed in the hairdresser's, crawled home and lost consciousness for about four hours. When she came to, her whole body hurt and she had pins and needles all over. The back of her head was tender and she felt severely depressed, which was unusual for her. Although she did not take any more pills she had continuous pain for the next two years and sometimes felt suicidal.

Later she had two pregnancies and suffered migraine throughout both. When her first son was born she was suddenly covered in a rash and after the second she bled from her breasts. By the time I saw Mrs YG she had been given a variety of drugs which were either useless or made her feel worse.

One of her sons was always needing antibiotics for very worrying upper respiratory infections. John was investigated at the Westminister Hospital Immunology Unit, the department where much of the early bone marrow work was pioneered. John's blood was completely lacking in immunoglobin A (IgA). This hereditary defect affects about one in a hundred people. There are four main immune proteins circulating in the blood — IgM, IgA, IgG and IgE. These antibodies are made by special white blood cells which originate from more primitive cells in the bone marrow. Newly born infants have hardly any immunoglobins in their blood and they rely heavily on their mothers' antibodies transferred in the milk. By the time children are seven years old, they usually have nearly the same immunoglobulin blood levels as adults. This is one reason young children are especially susceptible to infections. A few individuals, one or two in a hundred, have a hereditary IgA deficiency and they are particularly likely to have recurrent respiratory or gastro-intestinal infections. IgA is normally plentiful in the gut where food is broken down and absorbed. John's mother Mrs YG also had almost no IgA. They both had normal IgE levels.

We now know that daily exposure to cigarette smoke can precipitate hay fever or asthmatic attacks as well as migraine attacks and therefore may be a cause of raised IgE, but neither Mrs YG nor John were exposed to cigarette smoke.

Migraine and Allergy

Migraine was not thought to be due to allergy as there are exactly the same number of atopic individuals with raised IgE levels among migraine sufferers as there are in the general population. Nevertheless, because of Mrs YG's experiences, I wondered if immune abnormalities were the main cause of adverse reactions to times of hormone changes and drug treatments, so I asked for the serum immunoglobulins to be measured on all the migraine patients I saw. As IgE is present in the blood in very small amounts only IgM, and IgA and IgG are routinely investigated by hospital Chemical Pathology departments as these immunoglobulins can be altered in liver disease, cancer, especially myeloma and arthritis.

Most of our patients had values within the normal range but some had too high or low levels. Dr Bruce Müller continued this work for me at Charing Cross Hospital and we eventually discovered that when patients stopped the pill, avoided smoking, stopped ergotamine or changed their diet, their abnormal proteins levels significantly returned to within the normal range and they stopped having migraine attacks. The highest IgG levels (up to 2.3 grams/100mls) were reached by some heavily smoking men taking ergotamine.[4] A few patients like Mrs YG have a hereditary defect in IgA levels and these defects appear to be permanent, but mostly the antibodies change according to daily habits.

I had been using the 1972 Guildford normal values but I noticed that these normal ranges had widened seven years later at Charing Cross. I checked with various London hospitals. Each gave slightly different figures but all the 'normal' ranges had widened since 1972.

The hospitals had used samples of blood donated to the transfusion service. This blood is mostly given by young adults who are more likely to be smoking or taking the pill than the average person. We also gathered one hundred 'control' bloods from nurses and laboratory technicians but, again, most had smoked or taken the pill and many had headaches or allergies. However, larger scale studies carried out elsewhere showed clearly that either the pill alone or smoking alone can significantly alter immune proteins.

My paper at the 1974 migraine Trust Symposium[5] aroused the interest of a young Australian neurologist, Dr George

Lord. He was able to discover that some migraine patients had temporary immune changes in their blood at the onset of their headaches. One patient was so sensitive to the plant daphne, that after smelling its strong perfume, she produced immune complexes and had a migraine attack a few hours later. But mostly patients get migraine attacks after eating particular foods. Dr Hanington recorded that women were more likely to react to these foods before their periods or when they took the pill.

Oestrogenic Moulds

Migraine has been linked with reactions to food for hundreds or perhaps thousands of years. Primitive man for millions of years ate a stone age diet of fresh food consisting mostly of meat, fish, fruit and nuts. About ten thousand years ago the first settled communities appeared and wild grasses began to be cultivated as regular crops. The grains could be stored and ground into flour for making bread. Grains, however, can go mouldy and bread is leavened by yeast — also a fungus. One story of the earliest neurosurgery is that a hole was bored through the skull bone to let out evil spirits (or to relieve migraine?). Dr Gina Schoental of the Royal Veterinary College thinks that mycotoxins, common in grains, have always been a powerful cause of disease, especially those with actions like oestrogens.

Food Allergies

A Scottish doctor, Francis Hare, revived interest in food allergies at the beginning of this century when he wrote *Food Factor in Disease* in 1905, based on his meticulous work carried out in Australia. Dr Theron Randolph, the founder of modern Clinical Ecology, was inspired by the writings of Francis Hare and worked with Dr Albert Rowe, who introduced elimination and rotation diets. Dr Randolph was a physician in a hospital in Chicago when he recognised the importance of chemicals in our day-to-day environment at the start of an investigation of an allergic patient. Dr Randolph told me recently that early in his career he became appalled at the often permanent harm which was being caused by the widespread use of the new steroid wonder drugs. Cortisone, then later prednisone, were being given to arthritics to mask their pain and curb the inflammation but had serious long-term effects including permanently damaging the immune system. At a Clinical Ecology Conference in London in 1982, Dr Randolph said he completely agreed with me that no one should be given steroids. Steroids are used for emergency treatment, for example in neurosurgery, but Dr Randolph is completely against their unnecessary use.

Dr Randolph's new branch of medicine has been sweeping America, especially since the growing use of the pill in the sixties. The first symposium of the American Society of Clinical Ecologists was held in the British West Indies in 1966.

Meanwhile, a lone star had appeared in Britain — Dr Richard Mackarness, general practitioner, medical journalist and Clinical Assistant in Psychiatry at Park Prewett Hospital, Basingstoke. In 1958 he wrote his first bestseller *Eat Fat and Grow Thin*. He described how patients could diet by avoiding cereals and sugars, which were the main culprits, and he advocated a stone age diet. He met Dr Randolph that year and eventually produced *Not all in the Mind*[6] in 1976 which was quickly followed by *Chemical Victims*. Unfortunately Dr Mackarness has now emigrated to Australia. His latest book, *A little of what you fancy*, is a very useful guide and help in giving up smoking and other addictions, including common foods. Before leaving he helped twelve of us found the British Society for Clinical Ecology. This rapidly enlarging society has many new members at each meeting; doctors dedicated to the idea that most common illnesses are caused by contact with substances in our daily environment. The answer to illness is not just symptomatic drug treatment but to find out the causes and try to avoid them.

When I first read a review of *Not all in the Mind* I was excited and phoned the author at once saying 'That's what the pill does — it causes food allergy'. I wondered if women made ill by the pill would get better if they followed an exclusion diet. Dr Mackarness was, at that time, advocating food testing after a complete fast for five days, eating nothing and only drinking spring water. I did not see how I could endure that, far less expect my migraine patients to cope with such an ordeal.

A few months went by and one of my patients, successfully weaned off ergotamine, but still having headaches, heard of Dr Mansfield, a Banstead general practitioner. He had adapted the Mackarness diet and his patients added lamb and fresh pears to the spring water, in glass bottles, for the first five days. I tried this diet myself and discovered that I reacted to tea, oranges, yeast tablets, mushrooms and bread. After this I was sold on Clinical Ecology. I have advised nearly all the patients I have seen since to try the diet as a first step in a diagnosis and treatment. The results are quite amazing. Each patient found out which foods were troublesome and severe migraine attacks and high blood pressure became a thing of the past. Even bad skin rashes disappeared.

Rotation Diet

It isn't simply a matter of eliminating toxic food however, as Dr Randolph discovered when he wrote *Human Susceptibility to the Chemical Environment* in 1958.[7] Not only are people more likely to damage their natural immune mechanisms if they take daily drugs or steroids, like the pill, but daily exposure to chemicals like domestic gas and cigarette smoke are great hazards. Dr Randolph recommends alkalis, a weak solution of sodium or potassium bicarbonate, for quickly stopping a reaction to a food. Certain individuals, especially those prone to high blood pressure, are very sensitive to sodium bicarbonate and common salt, so they are better to use potassium bicarbonate alone. Some patients develop severe withdrawal symptoms when they stop their most frequently eaten foods or drinks and it is important that exclusion diets are carried out under medical supervision. Children, who react to fewer foods than adults, can start a four-day rotation diet at once. A different food should be eaten at each meal, e.g.: Day 1 — bananas, turkey, carrots; Day 2 — grapes, pork, green beans; Day 3 — pears, cod, potatoes; and Day 4 — rice, lamb, broccoli. This basic diet is continued while adding one new food each meal, leaving common allergens like milk, wheat and yeast till later.

I published the results of the first sixty patients who successfully completed the diet in the *Lancet* in May 1979.[8] In September, 1978, I had presented the results at an International Migraine Symposium in London. There was a great outcry. Some of the world's migraine experts found it hard to believe that sixty out of sixty patients stopped having migraine attacks — some for the first time in forty years — and most avoided even having headaches, all without taking any medication.

A typical patient was Mrs CE who was forty-seven and had taken the pill for eight years and prednisone for four years when I first saw her at the migraine clinic. She had a very thick hospital file, a relic of many visits and expensive investigations. Besides looking after her husband and children (one of whom was dyslexic) she was employed as a social worker. Her job involved being called out at night and she was finding her work an increasing burden. She was having nearly continuous headaches, frequent bouts of cystitis and arthritic pain in her left hip.

She had migraine since childhood and had always lived in a house with gas. She had smoked for twenty-seven years and had recurrent urinary infections for twenty-five

years. For the past four years she had been taking prednisone and antibiotics almost continuously but had added
leg cramps, tiredness, visual disturbances and arthritis to
her symptoms. I first asked her to discontinue the prednisone gradually and stop the pill and smoking. She was
much better but still had some headaches.

Mrs CE started the elimination diet on a caravan
holiday and went into a deep sleep probably because she
was allergic to both lamb and the calor gas in the caravan.
Her husband was also smoking. Back home, she tried
again with cod instead of lamb for the first five days. This
time she completed the diet and I published her results in
the *Lancet*. She had pulse rises when she ate beef, green
beans and milk and each gave her a headache and urinary
pain and frequency. Milk made her feel dizzy and pork
increased her pulse by 30 beats per minute and she felt
anxious. Bread made her feel sleepy. She also reacted to
chocolate, coffee, orange and mushrooms.

Her IgG and IgA were low (probably due to taking
steroids for so long). Her absorption and her liver function
were abnormally fast. She was very much better eating a
rotatory diet. Her headaches and cystitis had gone and,
although previously she had come near to losing her job,
she was now promoted at work.

A few patients react to everything on testing, especially
if they have been taking steroids and I think it is important
for them to rotate very strictly with a different food each
meal, provided the diet is nutritionally sound and the
patient does not lose weight. It is also of critical importance that gas, tobacco fumes and traffic fumes should be
avoided if possible. Mrs CE continued to work in busy
London streets but the other patient I described in the
Lancet, moved to a gas free house at the sea side where she
has remained free from headaches.

But they did not only stop having migraine. I listed the
other complaints of the first twenty-six patients and mood
changes had been even more common than headaches.

Tiredness	23	Hypertension	10
Depression	5	Obesity	10
PMT	15	Oedema	5
Violence	1	Cystitis	1
Ergot addiction	9	Colitis	1
Tobacco addiction	5	Constipation	4
Acne	1	Mastitis(breast lumps)	5
Painful periods	2	Fibroids	1

All these conditions improved or disappeared completely.

Mr Ian Burn, the consultant surgeon who runs Charing Cross's breast clinic said he's never seen lumps disappear so quickly. Even the fibroids disappeared before the planned operation. Since then Mr Burn has advised his lady patients to stop smoking as well as stop taking the pill and he has cut down the number of diagnostic biopsy operations. This is similar to the Gentle Method of cancer treatment which allows an excellent diet with mineral and vitamin supplements to strengthen the body's immune system so that it can cope with the disease.

It is easy to tell if patients are sticking to a good rotation diet and avoiding their allergens, especially yeast. They become their correct weight and have a bright, shiny look. Dark circles round the eyes are an excellent indicator that troublesome foods and chemicals are not being avoided.

I also listed the commonest foods causing reactions among sixty patients.

	%		%
Wheat	78	Beef	35
Orange	65	Corn	33
Eggs	45	Cane-sugar	33
Tea	40	Yeast	33
Coffee	40	Mushroom	30
Chocolate	37	Peas	28
Milk	37		

These sixty patients had taken an average of 115 tablets each month before the diet but only half a tablet afterwards.

Another graph showed how older patients had more reactions as the number of foods causing reactions increases with age. Of the first sixty consecutive patients only eight were men and all the younger women, of which there were twenty-nine, had been using oral contraception for an average of three years. The smokers had smoked for an average of twenty years.

When I finished my lecture some experts at the symposium rushed up to the platform, took the microphone out of my hand and wanted to know more details about the immune mechanisms involved. Dr Lord, the Australian neurologist, later showed me his slides demonstrating the immune complex and complement changes at the onset of some migraine attacks but, at the time, I had not read his papers[9] and only knew what I had already said, that abnormally low or high total serum immunoglobulins G, A and M tended to return to normal and so I was unable to answer every question.

Food Antibodies

We had not measured total IgE. We had, however, the help of the most distinguished clinical immunologist Professor Jack Pepys of the Cardiothoracic Institute, Brompton Hospital, and his registrar. They had measured antibodies to six common foods — egg white and yolk, corn, wheat, milk, orange and coffee, using a technique called ELISA (enzyme linked isoabsorbent assay). Antibodies to these foods were carried by IgG and IgE proteins. Unfortunately, our results were not published, as Professor Pepys wanted me to find controls. How could I? I could hardly expect people with no complaints to eat lamb and pears for five days and give up tea and coffee for a week or two. I said 'What about your laboratory workers?' He said they wouldn't do as they were nearly all atopic (allergic). I was keen to find controls using the Bryan cytotoxic test when weak solutions of foods are added to live blood cells, changes in the white cells and platelets show if the patient is allergic. It is a quick and useful test for finding out if a person reacts to only a few foods or a great many although it is only 80 per cent reliable. [10] I was unable, therefore, to persuade the Professor of Haemotology at Charing Cross to organise this.

By this time, Amelia Nathan Hill, an early 'miraculously cured' migraine patient of Dr Mansfield's, had started 'Action Against Allergy'(AAA). Amelia had suffered from a lifetime of severe migraine and the world's migraine experts had been unable to help. She brought several of her AAA members, including her friend and secretary Aeronwy Ellis (Dylan Thomas' daughter), to see me at Charing Cross to have the latest tests done.

These included liver tests, absorption tests, glucose tolerance tests and tissue typing, such as is used in kidney or bone marrow transplants, to see if migraine or allergic patients had a particular hereditary white cell typing (like ABO red cell blood groups). We did not find any one particular marking such as has been found with some, usually rare diseases, but we did find that two of our worst patients who reacted to everything with unusual severity, each had 'super slow' markers; two in fifty patients was more than expected. Again, this study was not published as the immunologist Dr Bill Ollier wanted to test a larger sample.

When Aeronwy Ellis' food-blood result came back she had the highest antibody levels to milk out of fifty and the second highest to egg. She was pregnant at the time and had just been admitted to a local hospital because of bleeding from her stomach. She was given only a 40 per cent chance of living. When Aeronwy heard of her high antibody levels to milk, she told us she had been drinking a pint of milk a day during the pregnancy. She avoided these foods for the rest of her pregnancy, making a dramatic recovery and after a few more months gave birth to a healthy, normal daughter. Aeronwy had tried to take an oral contraceptive pill on five occasions. Twice she tried for a week but became dangerously suicidal. The other times she stopped after two days when she felt the nervousness and anxiety returning.

Food Allergies and Liver Function

We had found abnormally high or low antibody blood levels tended to return to the normal range when the pill was stopped, but this did not necessarily happen to pill-induced changes in liver function. The liver is a bag of enzymes. Food is broken down and digested in the gut and then transported in the blood stream to the liver. The liver enzymes convert carbohydrates into sugar, proteins into amino acids and fats into fatty acids. It also makes immune proteins — antibodies to circulate in the blood stream. Routine hospital tests are rather insensitive and mostly indicate liver cell damage such as happens in viral hepatitis or alcoholism. When a more sensitive test was developed it was soon found that oral contraceptives tend to slow down the action of one of the main detoxifying enzymes aryl hydrocarbon hydroxylase (AHH), which deals with carcinogens such as petrochemicals, by as much as a third.

This test, known as the antipyrine clearance test, consists of measuring samples of blood or spit at three hourly intervals for 12 hours. The time the liver takes to metabolise a fixed dose of antipyrine is calculated. Normally the liver metabolises this drug in 20 to 28 hours. With the help of Dr Ifor Capel and his team from the Marie Curie Memorial Laboratories at Oxted, Surrey, we were able to test migraine patients at Charing Cross Hospital. Most of the younger women tested had been taking the pill and had abnormal liver function. Those with anorexia (bouts of refusing to eat followed by bouts of overeating and bingeing) tended to have very fast liver function and they had usually smoked as well as taken the pill. The more overweight ladies tended to have very slow function. Our results[11] varied from 'half lives' for antipyrine from 5 hours to over 32 hours, the normal range being 10 to 14 hours. Those with the most abnormal function, either too fast or too slow, had the most severe reactions to foods and chemicals.

Some reacted to everything they tested and suffered from what has been called the total allergy syndrome and were 'allergic to the twentieth-century'. It is tragic that these women, usually young women who have taken the pill, are often regarded as suffering from imaginary hysterical illness. When I persuaded the special metabolic ward at Charing Cross Hospital to admit and provide a diet for one of these patients while she had investigations, including liver function, there was a complaint from one of the nursing staff that the bed should be used by someone really ill. The result of the test came back as one of our most abnormal.

There is a great confusion in many people's minds, both medical and non-medical, about the overlap between mental and physical symptoms. When apparently healthy young men suddenly have heart attacks it is said to be because they have been suffering from 'stress'. The stress mechanisms are usually perfectly well able to cope with much more stress than people think, provided they are not compromised by too much alcohol, tobacco smoking, pollution by chemicals, and above all by the use of steroids such as the pill, which alter the body's regulating mechanisms.

We found that most of our patients with numerous allergies also had abnormal absorption rates and glucose tolerance tests. It is known that allergy to gluten in wheat, oats and rye can cause the intestinal villi to atrophy, which in turn increases the absorption of abnormally large particles of food in the blood stream. Tea and coffee speed up liver function and interfere with normal absorption as does alcohol drinking and cigarette smoking.

Alcoholism

Not only is alcohol a brain and liver poison but most alcoholic drinks are made from common allergens such as yeast and grains. Their absorption can be speeded up so much that alcoholic beverages have been described as 'delivering allergens with the speed of a jet-propelled vehicle'. Many women taking the pill notice they are more likely to have hangovers if they drink but, perhaps because allergy and addiction are closely interlinked, there has been a huge increase in the number of young alcoholic women in recent years. Women now outnumber men in some London alcoholic treatment centres, and women, especially if they also take the pill, are more likely to sustain serious liver damage compared with men. In 1966 the ratio of women to men alcoholics was estimated to be about one to eight. By 1976 this had arisen to one to three and by 1979 to almost one to one. The average age of women seeking help at Fulham Hospital in London has dropped from over fifty to between twenty-five and forty.

A recent survey of British women has also found that only 16.4 per cent were teetotal compared with 50 per cent in American studies. A Charing Cross Hospital survey found 58.1 per cent of women drank during pregnancy and a quarter of all women surveyed were moderate to heavy drinkers.[12]

Research into alcohol addiction has come up with an exciting theory which is also relevant for women made ill by taking the pill. (Alcohol levels may be 30 to 50 per cent higher in women who take the pill.)

Prostaglandins

The pill causes upsets in protein and fat metabolism and both of these can lead to distortions of prostaglandin metabolism. (See Chapter 3.) While amines were the focus of brain research in the sixties, the prostaglandins (PGEs) have been the interest of the seventies. (The name means glandular secretion of the prostate.) Semen contains a large amount of PGE_1, which, like amines, is an important mood regulator. Platelets from patients with depression make less PGE_1 than normal, while those from euphoric parents with mania make more than normal.

Dr David Horrobin has suggested that variations in PGE_1 levels may hold the key to alcohol addiction.[13] Although alcohol stimulates platelets to make PGE_1, it can also cause a shortage by blocking production at an earlier stage from the essential fatty acid — linoleic acid (LA). Even if an alcoholic is taking adequate amounts of vegetable oils containing LA, the individual will run short of PGE_1 and keep drinking more alcohol in order to feel good. Alcohol prevents LA being converted into GLA (Gamma-linolenic acid). But this block can be overcome by giving GLA in the form of an oil made from the seed of the evening primrose. The Latin name for the plant, *oenothera biennis*, means 'healer of the effects of wine'. Not only can a few drops of the oil prevent a morning hangover, but Doctors Iain and Evelyn Glen in Inverness have evidence that evening primrose oil significantly relieves alcohol withdrawal symptoms. Also in their tests abnormal liver enzyme levels returned to normal significantly faster than in their control group.

This story is connected with Professor Pfeiffer's discovery that people who suffer from mental illnesses tend to have higher levels of copper and low levels of zinc. The normal conversion of LA to GLA needs an adequate amount of zinc and vitamins.

Professor Guy Abraham summarised the literature on premenstrual tension[14] and noted that minerals such as calcium and magnesium were used as supplements to treat the condition as early as 1931. The most recent research suggests that women with severe PMS symptoms have prostaglandin imbalance, exaggerated reactions to hormones, and are likely to have correspondingly severe vitamin and mineral upsets. The correct supplements can be of great benefit in helping women recover from the pill, and such advice is essential before they become pregnant as I shall describe in Chapter 8.

Addiction

The more allergic a person becomes, the more addicted they become to stimulants and common social habits like smoking and drinking.

Mrs AM came to see me when she was thirty-seven. She had fairly frequent childhood infections and her father smoked a pipe. She did well at school and passed 'A' level Maths and Physics. She was given a job in a new computer firm and gained rapid promotion. She began smoking at nineteen and smoked up to thirty cigarettes a day for four years. She started taking contraceptive pills at twenty-four and continued with them for eight years in spite of being admitted four times to hospital for headaches and depression. She attempted suicide 'lots of times' by taking overdoses of her antidepressant medication.

When When Mrs AM first took the pill she noticed she became depressed. Her doctor said it was nerves because she was about to be married. She stopped the pill for a month or two but as she still felt depressed, she started taking it again. From the age of nineteen to thirty, she drank two or three whiskies a day. She became severely allergic to certain foods, to fumes and moulds. Exposure to domestic gas made her faint. She was complaining of exhaustion, being suicidally depressed, attacks of loss of memory, headaches, nausea, dizziness, rashes, chest pains and feelings of being very cold or very hot. Her liver function test result was abnormally fast.

She had tried an exclusion and rotating diet. She had been desensitised to individual foods and chemicals but she deteriorated. She moved to a fume-free house in the country. Her marriage was broken and she had been unable to work for years. She has since been benefited by mineral and vitamin supplements and a three monthly desensitisation treatment. Although she had a serious reaction to the second treatment, she has been able to start full time work again after years of illness and is now well.

Action Against Allergy (AAA) has received thousands of similar requests for help. Many of the women tell about their suicide attempts when they were taking the pill.

In 1978, however, the medical establishment was not ready to accept the full implications of my results. People still remain sceptical now and many migraine experts continue to look for drug solutions. There is a general belief that it is possible to go on smoking, drinking and taking the pill, and then take a magic drug which will miraculously make everything all right.

Meanwhile, Clinical Ecology in Britain has gone from strength to strength. More and more doctors are asking their patients to stop smoking and are giving diet sheets instead of writing prescriptions. They are finding their drug bill drops precipitously. In view of this, I wonder, how much of the National Health Service drug bill of over one and a half billion pounds each year is really necessary or beneficial. Some clinical ecologists find they have to give up NHS general practice. They only see private patients so that they can afford to spend enough time with each patient, but often only two or three visits are necessary compared with years of hospital attendance. At least one GP has remained in the NHS, however, and his drug bill is now so low that he is able to prescribe minerals and the DHSS is very interested in what he has been able to achieve.

Immune Changes

In 1969, an editorial in the *Journal of the American Medical Association* warned doctors to be on the alert for signs of oral contraceptive steroid pills interfering with immune responses.[15] Progestogens, especially, were likely to cause auto-immune disease. Since then, multiple sclerosis has increased twice as much in women as in men.

In 1971, Joshi and others found that some women taking the pill were less able to form antibodies.[16] In 1972, Hagen and Froland described how white cells from pill-taking woman reacted abnormally to testing with PHA (phyto-haemagglutinin).[17] The consultant physician, Dr Ronald Finn, who later proved to the *Lancet*'s satisfaction, by a double blind trial, that headaches could be caused by coffee addiction, and who is now the secretary of our British Society for Clinical Ecology, looked at those lymphocytes down the microscope and asked himself what chaos it was going to cause. His reaction was quite different from that of the Royal College of General Practitioners. In their 1974 oral contraceptive study report they found significant increases in traditional allergic conditions and bacterial and viral infections. They quoted papers demonstrating that the pill steroids decreased antibody formation in rats, rabbits, mice and women. They concluded that the pill might suppress immunity but said 'the effect of such a suppression, if it exists, is unlikely to be of clinical importance'.

In the same year a French allergist, Dr Falliers, wrote to the *Lancet* to report several cases of severe pill induced allergies which disappeared when the pill was discontinued. But he wrote 'it must be remembered that in clinical medicine, once the fire is lit, removal of the match does not necessarily extinguish the flame'.

In 1979, another French doctor, Dr J. L. Beaumont, and his team discovered a possible immunological basis for this view. They found that one in three women taking the pill had immune complexes containing antibodies to ethinyl oestradiol (the oestrogen in all the combined pills). The women who had developed thrombosis or phlebitis had the highest oestrogen antibody levels. The antibodies could be found two months after the pill was started and they persisted for years after the pill was discontinued as an 'immunological scar'.[18]

Dr Bill Rea, a cardiovascular surgeon who runs a clinical ecology unit in Dallas, reports causes of persistent, recurrent thrombophlebitis, and 85 per cent of these patients are women.

The most difficult patients to put right are women who

have been using the pill for years, especially if they have continued in spite of warning symptoms.

Mrs SL came to consult me recently because of feeling unwell for the past ten years. She said she had always been fit as a child. She had an identical twin sister, but Mrs SL was the healthier of the two and was hardly ever ill.

In 1967 she began to take a contraceptive pill, which she took for eight years from the age of twenty-three to thirty-one. During this time she gradually and insidiously became ill. She was getting headaches, disliked gas and petrol fumes, felt tired, depressed and anxious, especially at period times. She stopped taking the pill seven years ago but did not start to feel better. She had rashes and her hands became swollen. She reacted to sunlight. She had breast lumps. She was now reacting to many different foods and had difficulty carrying out an exclusion and rotating diet. Her twin sister, who had never taken the pill, feels perfectly well and is now the fitter of the two.

After the Pill

There are various approaches being tried for patients who lack the will power or the ability to stick to a rotation diet which includes a wide variety of foods.

Desensitisation

This approach is immunological. Attempts are made to desensitise patients to common foods.[19] A food is diluted until only a trace exists in different solutions. These are dropped under the tongue in sublinqual provocation tests, or injected into the skin. The exact dose causing symptoms is noted and the nearest dose which makes the symptoms and signs disappear is found. The patient is given this neutralising dose to take or inject daily. Attempts, using the same technique have been made to neutralise against hormones —

oestrogens and progesterones. The American paediatrician, Dr Doris Rapp, shows a film of one of her patients who had become wild and violent when taking oestrogen. Dr Rapp gives the girl a neutralising injection and the pill patient immediately recovers. Dr Rapp's double blind tests are difficult to refute, but it is perhaps doubtful whether the neutralising approach is really the best for long-term management.

Nutrition

We found that the patients with the most numerous food reactions were most likely to have high blood copper and low blood zinc levels. High toxic metals and deficiencies of essential metals have become very common as are deficiencies or excesses of vitamins. These can be measured and supplements given as I shall describe in Chapter 8. The correct diet and nutrition can dramatically improve patients with multiple reactions to foods and chemicals.

Yeast Connection

The treatment of candida, momlia or thrush involves the prescription of an antifungal antibiotic like nystatin, while the patient eats a low carbohydrate diet and avoids foods containing sugar and yeast. It is thought that yeast infestation of the gut is a major cause of multiple sensitivities.[20] Progestogens dry up vaginal secretions, and vaginal infections, — whether herpes, gonorrhoea, thrush or trichomonas — and are more likely to be a problem among pill users. Herpes and thrush can adversely affect new-born babies if their mothers have not been treated before becoming pregnant.

Steroid users are also more likely to be given repeated courses of antibiotics which kill off the usual gut bacterial flora, allowing an overgrowth of thrush in the bowel. Although vitamin B_6 can benefit some women with pill-induced depression and premenstrual tension, patients with a strong yeast allergy are unable to tolerate many multi-vitamin B preparations if they have been made from yeast. Specially prepared low allergy vitamin pills are necessary.

Diet, supplements and nystatin may be very useful for highly sensitive patients with yeast allergies and may give dramatic results. Special care is needed, however, for women who are trying to become pregnant as it is best they avoid any medication during pregnancy. Mothers-to-be should try to regain their health before they attempt to conceive.

Fertility

Normally about 14 per cent of couples have trouble conceiving and a substantial number of women are unable to become pregnant after they stop the pill. In about one in 200 women brain hormones or ovaries having been articially blocked by the pill hormones, refuse to start working again automatically. It has been calculated that for most women fertility returns to normal within two years but only, in many cases, after they have had extensive investigations and courses of stimulating hormone treatments.

When human chorionic gonadotrophine (hCG) is used to stimulate the ovaries, one in five women have multiple births. When a LH luteinising hormone stimulating hormone is given this risk is avoided.[21]

Foresight, the Association for Pre-conceptual Care, has found that many infertile couples benefit from diet, mineral and vitamin supplements and avoiding common social poisons. I think these simple methods should always be tried first before hormones are given. This is especially important for young girls with period problems. Some of my patients have found their periods became regular just by avoiding a few common foods.

Pesticides

Thanks to space research techniques, it is now possible to measure minute amounts of toxic chemicals such as parts per billion of chlorinated pesticides in our blood. Doctors running environmental units are becoming increasingly aware that sensitive women, who cannot tolerate pill hormones, have high levels of these toxic pesticides. Some of these pesticides, so commonly sprayed on cereals, fruit and vegetables, can interfere with our body's own hormones. It is ironic that antifungal agents are sprayed on stored grain to kill the oestrogenic mycotoxins when they in turn add to our body burden of harmful chemicals.

Summary

* The pill steroids drastically alter immune functions

* They increase both allergies and infections and there are multiple obvious or hidden (masked) reactions to foods and chemicals

* The cause severe vitamin and mineral imbalances and alterations to food absorption and liver function

* Antibodies to pill hormones can persist for years increasing the chance of further severe reactions

* Treatment can include exclusion, rotation stone-age diets and mineral and vitamin supplementation, treatment of yeast allergy and occasionally neutralisation and use of environmental units for severe cases.

6   Trial and Error

Common belief: *In pill trials women who are on the pill are compared to women who are not.*

Fact: *Many 'control' women have been prescribed hormones for gynaecological problems.*

There is nothing more likely to perplex the woman on the pill than turning for guidance to scientific trials and studies which have attempted to evaluate the safety of her contraception. There have been a number of these carried out mainly over the past decade and some of them have produced evidence to suggest that the pill confers some health benefits on those who take it. I believe these claims to be unfortunate, and responsible for diverting attention from the huge rise in cancer, especially in younger women.

Statistical evidence is the sacred end result of properly conducted studies but statistics can be misleading. Confusing conclusions, however, so common in the pill controversy, are the result of the difficulty in comparing all the variables so that the truth is clear. For example, in order to compare women on the pill with 'control' women who are not, it would be necessary to recruit controls whose bodies have not been exposed to steroid hormones. This does not always happen. In the big American Walnut Creek study it was reported that women over forty who had never taken the pill were significantly more likely to have endometrial cancer than those who had — yet of the 3,947 women in the 'never-user' group 1,263 had taken oestrogens! Oestrogen use at any time, past or present, significantly increased the risk of this type of cancer in women over fifty.[1]

The confusion here can be blamed on a fashion for prescribing hormones whenever a woman of any age presents herself to her doctor with period or menopausal problems. These seem to be the lazy answer to 'women's troubles' and, because of this, many women have been 'on the pill' without being aware of it. In most American studies 80 per cent of women under forty have used the pill, and depending on the centre, between 10 to 50 per cent of forty to sixty year olds have used hormones. It would be more helpful in large pill studies if there was a separate category into which women who have been treated for gynaecological problems with steroid hormones could go, although nowadays such women are given combined or sequential pills like oral contraceptive users as oestrogens alone are considered too dangerous. And, this is in spite of the fact that the pill was thought to be too dangerous for women over thirty-five

However, because so many women take part in these studies, it is almost impossible to get the full facts about them. If their GP has made any special selection regarding them, perhaps refraining from giving them the pill because of a suspected or inherited medical condition, the reason is not always known by those conducting the trials and inevitably the results are affected. If a woman with a predisposition to an illness, such as rheumatoid arthritis, is prevented from going on the pill by her doctor, and entered into a trial as a non-user control, and a woman with a strong immunological system who stays on the pill without serious side-effects goes into that study, then the potential for claiming pill-benefits can be guessed. I am not suggesting that this is something which is calculated in any way but merely pointing to the natural bias which can enter trials. And yet these appear as foolproof evidence when presented to the public.

It is my experience that it is the stalwarts who stay on the pill, those women who are super-strong and can withstand the steroid onslaught for much longer than women whose bodies have reacted fast and stopped them endangering their health with oral contraceptives. I believe it is this fact which will always give an unbalanced picture in the results of trials, for they will be studying many women whose health is basically sound, and who have excellent defence systems.

There are also the big gaps left by doctors and patients who don't report specific side-effects. I've seen numerous patients who think they have had no side-effects with the pill because they have been told by their doctors that their complaints and symptoms are unrelated or they did not think themselves that they were related. Even I did not connect my own leg symptoms with the pill until my husband suggested it.

Higher rates of illness in women who have stopped the pill are sometimes used to show that current users are protected from some of the ill health — but I think this merely shows that the current users' tolerance has not yet expired. In 1968 two large scale trials were started, the Royal College of General Practitioners Oral Contraceptive Study[2] — enrolling 47,174 women between 1968 and 1969, and the Oxford/FPA study[3] enrolling 17,032 women during 1968 and 1974. In both cases half the women were enrolled as controls using other methods of birth control, although some of them switched over to the pill and were entered as takers. Women who already had illnesses known to be made worse by the pill were likely to be in the control or non-user group — so the pill women were healthier at the start than the control women.

RCGP Study

In the first results of the RCGP study it was shown that very few new pill users were still on it by their third year. Most had stopped the pill because of side-effects or they had been lost to follow up by the researchers. By 1979, only a small percentage of the 23,378 women originally enrolled were known to be still using the pill — even allowing for the fact that they could stop and restart after a pregnancy. Six

105

out of ten women had been lost, and of the rest most changed to another method before the end of three years. Over 6,000 control women had been changed into the pill taking group helping to boost the rapidly dwindling number of pill users.

When a review of the first few years of the study was published in 1974[2], the commonest single cause of death among pill takers was suicide, which accounted for the death of nine women. Although the control women had suffered more illnesses before they were enrolled into the study, only four of them were known to have committed suicide. Altogether there were nineteen violent deaths among pill takers but only six among women using other methods. And these figures do not take into account that already 13,490 women could not be traced including 1,636 more pill takers than controls.

The big exodus was hardly surprising as the 1974 report showed that a large number of medical conditions were increased in pill users. Thrombosis was increased six times (although also reduced by a quarter with the lower doses of oestrogen). Strokes were increased four times, headaches three times, migraine and high blood pressure twice. There were large increases in many infections, vaginal discharges and cervical erosions. The occurrence of some allergic conditions too was shown to be significantly increased, and the report also showed there were possible increases in coronary artery disease, gall bladder disease, nasal catarrh, allergic rhinitis, hay fever, ulcerative colitis, Crohn's disease, virus diseases, pleurisy, epilepsy and schizophrenia. On stopping the pill sudden episodes of schizophrenia could occur because discontinuing steroids alters the body's own steroid production, which can make brain cells swell up with fluid, causing anxiety or other symptoms. This is called steroid withdrawal. These cases, described as early as 1967, see *Pill on Trial*[4] by Paul Vaughan, are unusual as only about one in a hundred people have a tendency to schizophrenia. I was discussing pill withdrawal causing illness with a colleague, however, when she suddenly realised this was what had happened to her daughter.

Sarah had been on the pill for several years. One day a nurse friend was telling her that there were several very ill young women in her ward suffering from thrombosis and she said she didn't know why the government allowed the pill to be prescribed as it seemed to be causing too much illness. This conversation prompted Sarah to stop taking the pill. She started to work harder and harder and progressively became more and more anxious. She thought she had to do all the work for the firm by herself and often worked very late. Her mother thought she was behaving strangely for several days, then Sarah completely lost touch with reality. She was admitted to hospital and was unable to work for the next six months. Since then she has made an excellent recovery.

By 1979 the women had been observed for ten years[5], fifteen pill users had committed suicide compared with seven in the control group. There were also twice as many deaths from accidents among pill users. All deaths from violence now totalled thirty-four and seventeen respectively.

These figures may underestimate the real risk as among the women followed up nearly half had stopped taking the pill within the first two or three years of the study, although thousands still wished to use contraception and the commonest illness among the two hundred different ones reported during their month of stopping the pill was 'neurotic depression'. Altogether, mental illnesses were reported twice as often as headaches and migraine during the last month.

The 1974 report summarised the 'adverse and beneficial association' with the pill in a simple diagram. The enormous increase in 'adverse' effects — migraine, vaginal discharge, depression, viral infections and loss of libido were shown in long stippled columns labelled 'subject to substantial bias'. The commonest 'beneficial' associations, listed as improving menstrual disorders and iron deficiency anaemia, were shown in short, solid columns labelled 'probable', giving the impression they were real benefits and not merely the inevitable consequences of taking a progestogen, which atrophies the lining of the womb and causes depression. By listing most of the illnesses caused by the pill as 'substantially biased', as if women were exaggerating their side-effects, the Royal College may have helped to give the impression that the pill has more benefits than disadvantages. In fact, the study found a *significant increase in over sixty conditions*. Against such a catalogue of serious illness in previously healthy young women, the benefits were said to be less bleeding from the dried up lining of the womb, less premenstrual tension — even though the mood effects were now continuous in many women instead of a few days before a period — and less breast disease, although the women who gave up had more breast disease than women who had never taken the pill. High doses of progestogen and longer pill use was claimed to be especially protective but only 3,731 women-years of use were recorded with high doses compared with 22,513 women-years on lower doses.

The conclusions of the 1974 report were summarised like this:

> Oral contraceptive users report an average of six episodes of illness every three years while non-users report an average of five episodes every three years. The additional episode in pill users is almost certainly not caused by the pill, but results from biased reporting associated with pill usage.

From their results the College expected some health benefits would be common, while adverse effects were rare. Although new risks might appear after longer observation, their evidence suggested that women could take the pill for longer and reduce the number of unplanned pregnancies.

These optimistic conclusions emerged in the press as 'Pill Gets All Clear'.

I wrote to the *British Medical Journal*[6] to complain that the high drop-out and side-effect rates did not justify the further use of the pill, but my detailed review was cut down to a short letter. Dr Valerie Beral, an Australian epidemiologist, who had noticed that more young women in Australia were dying of heart attacks since the pill was introduced, wrote to the *Lancet*.[7] She said it was a cause for concern that *women who had ever taken the pill had 39 per cent more chance* of dying of vascular disease or suicide from these figures. By 1977, Dr Beral had increased her estimate from further RCGP data — women who had *ever taken the pill were now four times (400 per cent)* more likely to die of cardiovascular disease and this risk was increased with age, especially for those over thiry-five years old (four out of every five women who had died of CV disease were over thirty-five), who smoked, and had more than five years of pill use.[8]

Curious Differences

In a review of many international controlled pill studies for the *British Journal of Family Planning* in 1980[9], Professor Martin Vessey discussed the increased risks of serious vascular diseases which were:

	Range	Average
Venous thromboembolism	1.5 to 11	×9
Thrombolic stroke	2 to 26	×6
Haemorrhagic stroke	—	×2
Subarachnoid haemorrhage	2 to 22	×6
Myocardial infarction	1 to 14	×4

There were very large differences of incidence given in different reports. These discrepancies obviously depend on the accuracy of the follow-up, the ages women are given the pill, their smoking habits and who are chosen as 'controls'. The only true controls would be healthy, non-smoking women who had never taken any type of pill steroid, but such women are becoming increasingly hard to find.

Death rates per 100,000 women years in women in the pill-taking age group

	England & Wales 1975	Oxford/FPA OC users at entry 1968-79	R.C.G.P. Ever users 1968-79	Walnut Creek All women % 1968-77
All deaths	108.5	52.9	87.2	100
Neoplasms	44.3	25.3	30	45
Circulatory	21.9	12.3	29.9	15
Accidents + Violence	17.1	4.6	18.2	19
Follow-up			42%	86.2%

Figure 3

Perhaps the most curious differences come with the causes of death in the three large pill studies — The Oxford/FPA study, the RCGP study and the Walnut Creek study. Professor Vessey has estimated the mortality rate for pill-taking age women in England and Wales in 1975 to be 108.3 per 100,000 women-years. The commonest cause of death was neoplasms at 44.3, with circulatory deaths half as likely at 21.9 and accidental and violent deaths third at 17.1

After ten years the women pill-takers enrolled in the Oxford/FPA study[10] recorded only half as many deaths as women in the country as a whole (52.9). They were twice as likely to have died of cancer (25.3) than vascular diseases (12.3) but their rate for accidents and violence was surprisingly low at 4.6, considering the study had found pill users to be four times more likely to make suicide attempts than diaphragm users.

Pill users in the RCGP study[5] also had a lower mortality rate (87.7) but here the main difference was that they had an equal risk of cancer (30) as circulatory death (29.9). Perhaps this apparent under-recording of neoplasms is because more than half the women in the study were never traced.

In the American Walnut Creek study 16,638 women aged

110

eighteen to fifty-four were enrolled between 1968 and 1972 but most of the 10,135 pill takers had started it during the previous six or more years and only 4,588 were still on it at the start of the study. When enrolled, these 'ever' users were significantly more likely to be taking tranquillisers or other medication and already had a higher incidence of over thirty-four medical ailments. One in ten of the pill users had also taken oestrogens and one in five of the 6,503 'never user' control women had also taken oestrogens.

After the ten years of the study, 13.8 per cent of the women were lost to follow-up. The remainder chalked up significant increases in cervical, breast and endometrial cancers if they had ever taken hormones (see Chapter 7). They also had increases in malignant melanoma, and lung cancer if they smoked as well. All six cases of urinary tract neoplasms and six of the seven thyroid cancers were in the pill users group. It is well-known that the pill can induce liver cancer but these tumours are too rare to show up in these relatively small studies.

During the ten years of observation there were 200 deaths but thirty were excluded from the final analysis because they were thought to be due to pre-existing conditions, thus dismissing the tumour-promoting effect of hormones. Of the remaining 170 deaths, 45 per cent were due to neoplasms which, in this study, were three times more common than circulatory deaths (15 per cent). Accidents and violence were second commonest at 19 per cent.

All three studies tended to exclude the most sensitive women at enrolment — those more likely to have side-effects and give up the pill within a month or two. In the Oxford/FPA study only women who had already continued with the pill for at least five months were chosen. Significantly fewer women with breast lumps were enrolled and pill users were eight times less likely to have had a history of previous thromboembolic disease than women using other methods. In the RCGP study only one in five women was a new pill taker; the others had already totalled 25,590

111

women-years of pill use and were obviously the tough survivors of a much larger number of women who had tried the pill during the previous four or five years.

An optimistic view of pill risks can result from starting with healthy, higher social class women who are kept well supervised, but it does not always help:

In 1978, Mrs Judith Challenger woke up one morning to find she was unable to move her left arm and leg. She had been a normal, healthy mother of two children who was also teaching. She had been taking a so-called 'low dose' pill for five or six years and had no symptoms other than some vague pains in face and nasal stuffiness which was diagnosed as sinusitis. She had recently been to her general practitioner for her regular six monthly check up. She asked her doctor if she should stop the pill, as she was now thirty-eight years old and she had read about the increased risk for those over thirty-five. He replied that her blood pressure and examination were normal and there was no reason why she should not continue on the pill until she was forty. In fact he said she was safer on the pill than driving to his surgery, which happened to be two miles away down a quiet country lane. Her doctor had believed that road accident fatalities were commoner than pill deaths. But women taking the pill are more likely to have accidents than others. Women are normally at maximum risk of having accidents during the few days before their period. With the pill this phase is prolonged from a few days to as much as twenty days.

Six weeks later, she was admitted as an emergency to hospital where a brain scan revealed a clot near the middle of the right side of her brain. She was able to move her leg after two weeks, her arm after several months and her hand after nine months. She still has some weakness in her left side and walks with a limp.

Mrs Challenger was determined to prevent this happening to other unsuspecting women and she started the Pill Victims Group. They have been gathering information and trying to gain compensation for the pill victims through the courts as has been done successfully in America on several occasions. In 1979, their lawyer, the American Gerald Sterns, went on British television and compared the detailed warning supplied with the pill in America with the scanty information given out with British pills. Within a month or two, new, detailed leaflets were being inserted in British pill packets. Following newspaper articles about the Pill Victims Group over seven hundred women (or their husbands if the wives were unable to write) wrote to Mrs Challenger. Most had had vascular disasters. Some women needed amputations, and others committed suicide because of their disabilities. She also has records of several cases of infertility due to amenorrhoea or, in a few cases, pituitary tumours. These tumours were very rare before the pill but are now more common. Perhaps the most distressing letter she received, however, was the one about a girl who was fifteen when she had her stroke. Mrs Challenger found that many of the pill victims had been prescribed the pill by doctors for medical or gynaecological reasons. It is common for teenage girls who are working hard for exams or are away from home for the first time to have irregular menstrual cycles and all too often the first line of treatment is hormones. In my experience, the best treatment is to follow a rotating low allergy diet and to avoid smoking.

Summary

* The pill increases death risk from all the main causes including cancer and vascular disease

* There are increases of most known illnesses among users and ex-users of the pill

* The pill does not prevent illness but may suppress symptoms

* The pill reduces period pain because no ovulation takes place

* The pill reduces monthly bleeding because progestogen causes atrophy (shrinking of the lining of the womb).

* Atrophy of the womb and ovaries means the cancer is increased, not deceased as is claimed.

7   Cancer and the Pill

Common belief: *Most pill deaths are due to circulatory disease*

Fact: *Women in the twenty-five to fifty age group are twice as likely to die from cancer.*

Does the pill cause cancer? This issue has split the medical world, creating a controversy which is truly alarming for women. It is a disturbing story which has not yet reached its climax and women are captive to the continuing studies which both confirm and deny the feared link.

The use of hormones has effectively put us all in danger. There are the 'DES sons and daughters' in America whose mothers were given diethyl stilboestrol (DES) during pregnancy, and who suffered reproductive organ cancers; there is the rise in cancers of the cervix and breast, especially in pill-taking countries, and there is the continued use of hormones in animal production which puts a question mark over our food.

When I began to give the pill in 1961 we knew that oestrogens caused cancer in animals but we were also giving 'protective' progestogens. The impression that progestogens protected against cancer came from their action on the lining of the womb. Oestrogen stimulates the gland cells to grow and divide rapidly. Prolonged oestrogen treatment causes a wild overgrowth of 'hyperplastic and cystic' glands. Sometimes the normal dividing mechanisms go berserk and the cells become malignant. But if enough progestogen is given the lining of the womb shrinks and disappears. Then, during the sixties, the pure progestogens such as chlormadinone and megestrol acetate were withdrawn because they were causing malignant breast lumps in dogs. MPA, another progesterone derivative which is in Depo-Provera has caused malignant womb cancers in monkeys and is suspected of causing cervical cancer in women.[1] To those of us who have become accustomed to hearing from the RCGP study that women who have ever taken the pill have a higher death rate, mostly due to a four times increase in circulatory disease, it comes as a surprise to learn that women in the twenty-five to fifty age group are in fact more than twice as likely to die from cancer as vascular disease.

Among our first 200 enrolled patients in the early London trials we had one case of breast cancer.

Mrs JL was thirty-five when she was given a sequential oral contraceptive — oestrogen only for fifteen days and both hormones for the next five days. Before starting the pill she noticed that her breasts were sore and lumpy before periods and she sometimes had migraine. After twenty months of this pill she was complaining of severe premenstrual tension with migraine and vomiting attacks. She had leg cramps at night, hot flushes and heavy withdrawal periods. I suggested she took the progestogen for ten days instead of five and Mrs JL felt much better. But six months later she' developed a hard lump in her left breast which was diagnosed as a rapidly growing cancer. Her long-term chance of survival was poor. In 1964 a woman of thirty-seven had a four in 10,000 chance of developing breast cancer. Had Mrs JL just been unlucky?

Mrs PD was one of the first patients enrolled at the Barnet clinic. She was in her early twenties and felt well on a combined pill. But after fourteen months she developed an extremely rare and highly malignant tumour in her thigh muscle — a sarcoma. Again, this could just have been bad luck, but the development of such rare and unusual cancers are now becoming news.

In the eighties we are seeing a unique type of sarcoma. In America young men of previously good health have been developing AIDS (acquired immune deficiency syndrome). The disease has been spreading at an alarming rate with over half dying within a year of diagnosis from either a wide range of viral, bacterial or fungal infections or from Kaposi's sarcoma. There is usually a history of over 1,000 different sexual partners before this serious illness develops.[2] The majority die within a year due to infection or the effects of the tumour. Before this current epidemic Kaposi's sarcoma mostly affected the skin of old men in Africa, and was rarely fatal. Testosterone levels fall in older men and they may become susceptible to their natural oestrogen production. AIDS is more common in passive homosexual partners[3] and many of these men take oestrogens. There is also another possible connection here. A study of young men whose mothers had taken oestrogen and progestogen during pregnancy has revealed that less than half were likely to be married, and the study group had a higher than normal incidence of sexual organ abnormalities. Men with abnormal testes are also more likely to develop testicular cancer — another increasingly common cancer.

The sarcoma affecting AIDS victims is a tumour of the blood vessels which spreads rapidly to skin and lymph organs. Post mortems of pill victims have shown similar blood vessel abnormalities and Dr Kitty Little saw a vascular tumour removed from a twenty-one-year-old girl which stretched the whole length of her largest artery. There is evidence that blood from individuals with AIDS can transmit the disease to haemophiliacs and other patients given blood transfusions, including in some cases a new born baby. This is a severe form of the immune changes I noticed in blood donated for transfusions. The so-called normal range for immune proteins has enlarged since the widespread use of the pill.

Cervical Cancer

By far the commonest type of cancer in young women which can be caused by the pill is cervical. In 1968, according to a report in *World Medicine*[4], two American studies had recorded a higher incidence of early cervical cancer, which is known as 'carcinoma in situ'. One study by Professor Weid estimated that the risk was increased six times from three in 1,000 to eighteen in 1,000 for those who had taken the pill for five years or more, although among 40,000 women screened only 500 were still using the pill after five years. The Weid study was never published as far as I know, but the other study by Melamed was published the following year.

At the same time I was finding that many of our pill takers had cervical erosions — large red, fleshy rough areas on the nect of the womb which bleed easily when you scrape them taking a cervical smear. These were especially common with high dose pills, whose high hormone levels particularly mimic the cell changes of pregnancy. Later, the RCGP study was to show that cervical erosions significantly increased with the dose of progestogen. Usually I sent the patients to have these healed by heat treatment and occasionally the women had to stop their pills to allow the cervix to heal naturally. One patient changed to half her previous dose after a six months' gap, but the erosion appeared once more. We did not have many cases of carcinoma in situ, but that may well have been because of our stringent monitoring of the women, who were examined every six months and treated promptly if lesions developed, and we had only a very small percentage who had taken the pill for five years or more.

Official registration for carcinoma in situ began in 1965. At that time a girl aged fifteen to twenty-four had a less than one in 100,000 chance of developing a positive smear. By 1978 the figures for England and Wales had increased ten fold from 0.8 per 100,000 to 8.5 per 100,000[5] and had increased by 1220% by 1981.

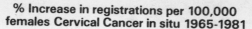

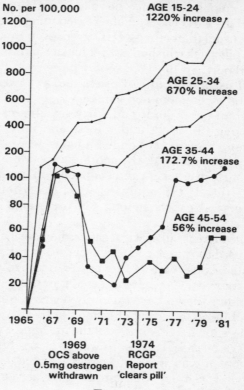

Figure 4

In 1972 very few single women in the country had ever used the pill (9 per cent) but by 1982 young unmarried girls made up the majority of first-time pill users at most clinics and the largest family planning clinic in Europe — the Margaret Pyke Centre in London — reported in the *Lancet* that one in twenty-five women attending had a positive smear and that there had been a sharp increase in serious forms.[6]

The Oxford/FPA study published in October 1983 said that all its sixteen cases of invasive cervical cancer had happened among women who had used the pill.[7] The numbers of the early cases had increased much more rapidly among pill users than among IUD users even though 28 per cent of the pill users who had not yet had a child were omitted from this report. In the 1978 report there were thirty cases among pill users, two in cap users, and yet twenty-one in smokers and eighteen in non-smokers.

The Walnut Creek study had thirty-seven cases of cervical cancer among pill users under forty and one case in the control group. Again, although smokers were statistically more likely to be affected, the actual figures were nearly the same — fourteen smokers and eighteen non-smokers.[8]

By 1983 the RCGP study reported thirty-four cases of invasive cervical cancer among pill users and ten among controls.[9]

While the increase in cervical cancer had been alarming, it has not caused too much concern because the early stages are easily treated. Nevertheless, the very low death rate in fifteen- to twenty-four year-olds has increased four times while death rates for older women have fallen by nearly a quarter.

Jean Robinson, a former chairman of the Patient's Association, has shown a link between the husband's occupation and the risk of cervical cancer as well as a possibly increased risk for women who work in textiles.[10] It has been known since the last century that nuns never develop cervical cancer, and well-known associations are age of first intercourse, multiple partners (incuding multiple partners of the male), venereal disease (especially herpes and genital warts), lower social class and folic acid deficiency. The sperm of lower-class, heavily smoking men may also cause cervical cancer. These sperm have an abnormal chemical structure — possibly due to lack of essential minerals like zinc and the presence of toxic metals like cadmium from smoking. As pill taking induces mineral and vitamin abnormalities in women, these could contribute to the increased risk of cervical cancer. It is, however, probable that women get cervical cancer from a combination of risk factors.

Until she reaches the age of nineteen, a woman's cervix lining is immature and especially susceptible to the changes that lead to malignancy. Every year younger than this that a girl starts to have sexual intercourse increases her risk of cervical cancer. The general availability of hot water, baths and showers should have helped to decrease the incidence of this disease but instead we have one in 100 pregnant women with a positive smear and many others who have had cervical operations before they have even become pregnant for the first time. It seems essential now to increase the frequency of cervical smear tests for women who have taken the pill but what is even more important is to discourage young women from going on it in the first place.

Dr Albert Singer said at a meeting of the Women's National Cancer Control Campaign (London, June, 1985) that a new incurable type of cervical cancer was becoming epidemic. The three year survival rate for women under 24 had declined from 93 per cent to only 72 per cent between 1977 and 1979. Half the under 40s inflicted with invasive cervical cancer now die within five years or less. When human papilloma virus type 16 was present in the man, eighty per cent of the women developed pre-cancerous smears. A 1985 WHO study from eight developing countries showed invasive cancer increased with length of pill use.

So much emphasis has been deliberately placed on greater sexual activity, especially numbers of partners and sexually transmitted disease, as a cause of cervical cancer that women are reluctant to admit their diagnosis to their family and friends. But the recent figures clearly show that the most important cause of invasive cancer in the young is taking the pill. Family planners are now tacitly admitting this by a campaign to increase the use of sheaths by men to protect their partners — this is the year (1985) of 'contraception for men'. Use of the sheath gives some protection from venereal diseases, but also protects against having to take the pill.

Breast Cancer

Over the past few years I have begun to feel that the establishment is ready to admit that oestrogen use causes cancer — it is difficult to deny it with endometrial cancer increasing six times (on average) in America through their increased use of oestrogens for menopausal symptoms.[11] But a rearguard action has been mounted. This has taken the line that progestogens are safe, but this diversionary tactic suffered a severe setback when Professor Malcolm Pike and his team from California presented his data in the *Lancet* in October 1983,[12] showing that breast cancer was increased four or five-fold among women who had taken the pill for six years or more before they were twenty-five, and the risk was greater for higher dose progestogen pills. It was the third study to find that young women who had begun the pill before they were twenty-five, or before their first full-term pregnancy, had an increased risk of breast cancer and the risk went up the longer the pill had been taken.

There was chaos, both in the medical world and the lay press, although it was now sixteen years since similar information had been available about cervical cancer. The appalling increase in cervical cancer had been efficiently blamed on sexual activity. But now in the same issue of the *Lancet*, the Oxford/FPA study results showed the pill was a main cause of cervical cancer to add to the breast cancer results.

Professor Pike's patients were Los Angeles County white women who had developed breast cancer between 1972 and 1982, and were younger than thirty-seven years old when diagnosed. Professor Pike told me that virtually all young women in California have tried the pill and 80 per cent had used it before they were twenty-five. He collected 510 cases of breast cancer, but fifty-two were already dead and the attending physicians refused permission to contact some of the others. Eventually 330 women with breast cancer completed the questionnaire and 314 matched for age and social class were found. The women with breast cancer had used the pill for longer — an average of 49.6 months compared with 39.2 months. But this was no new finding. Professor Sir Richard Doll and Professor Martin Vessey had published results in 1971[13] which found that more young women under forty with breast cancer had taken the pill for longer than two years compared with their controls — 50 per cent against 35.9 per cent — before the tumour was first noticed.

The opposite, however, was true for benign lumps — 62 per cent of users who developed lumps did so within their first year of pill taking. Only 14 per cent of the women with benign breast disease took the pill for more than two years compared with 33.3 per cent of the controls. This means that in on-going studies it seems that fewer women still taking the pill had breast disease compared with women using other methods of contraception. This started a very popular fashion for saying that the pill prevented benign breast disease. In fact their data had found fewer of these women had taken the pill for more than one year — 38 per cent compared with 59 per cent. But I think that this bears out what I have been saying all along — that the pill causes many symptoms, including breast lumps, in susceptible women so that they stop taking it. The most susceptible women tend to avoid breast cancer by giving up the pill after a few months while the tougher individuals stay on, symptom-free for years, unaware that they are increasing their cancer risk.

Professor Pike found twenty-four women with breast cancer had used a pill for more than seventy-three months before the age of twenty-five compared with only seven control women. Nine cancer cases had used what was called 'high' progestogen pills, but no control women had taken these common 'high' dose pills for so long. The conclusion was that 'low' progestogen pills 'appear to increase breast cancer risk little or not at all', but fifteen women with breast cancer had been long term users of these pills compared with seven controls — which seems more to me, however the statistics are calculated. Unfortunately Professor Pike and his colleagues had published a table giving values for oestrogen and progestogen potency of the oral contraceptives commonly used in the USA. The figures for oestrogen strength were simply based on the dose of oestrogen in micrograms in each pill. Mestranol was listed as having half the power of ethinyl oestradiol, e.g. 100 micrograms of mestranol was said to equal 50, while 50 micrograms of ethinyl oestradiol was also equal to 50. (Which makes nonsense of the original ban of any oestrogen dose of 50 micrograms because of thrombosis.)

The progestogen potency figures, ranging from 0.35 to 15, were taken from papers by Mishell and Greenblatt, which in turn were based on Dr Swyer's postponement of menstruation test. Dr Swyer had published this test in 1960, just before I joined him as an assistant.

Dr Swyer immediately wrote to the *Lancet* to challenge these 'progestogen potency' figures which, he said, took no account of the important combined effect of the oestrogen in the various combined pills.[14] He said his original test had in fact found only small differences between different progestogens, for example, norethisterone acetate had the same power to delay bleeding as ethynodiol diacetate. Their potencies were equal and not 2 to 15 as quoted by Professor Pike. Meanwhile the Committee on the Safety of Medicines had further confused the issue by hurriedly circulating British doctors with a list of figures for progestogen potency of British oral contraceptives which contained even more mistakes and misprints. These mistakes led to an unfortunate tendency to discredit the Pike paper which was entirely unfounded as far as his results that long-term pill use in young women could cause breast cancer were concerned. He had already stated in the paper that there were no good tests available to test the power of the hormones on breast tissue. He had definitely found an increased risk with the pills he had grouped as 'high' dose but his date of fifteen cases to seven controls for the 'lower' dose pills seems to me to show an increase with any type. It is difficult to understand the conclusion that low dose pills 'appear to increase the breast cancer risk little or not at all'.

In a further letter to the *Lancet* replying to questions about the safety of pills containing a low dose of oestrogen, Professor Pike and his colleagues stated that very few women in their study had used combined pills containing 35 micrograms or less of ethinyl oestradiol. Most who did used Lo/Ovral — 30 micrograms ethinyl oestradiol plus 0.3mg norgestrel, and among those four women with breast cancer had used Lo/Ovral for a total of 145 months. No controls had used that combination.

In December Dr Swyer wrote again to the *Lancet* to say that his delay of menstruation test relates only to a progestogen's ability to prevent bleeding and provides no evidence of the strength of its other actions. But if it did the range would be no more than 0.5 to 2.

Another letter to the *Lancet*[15] said that assessments of progestogen strength, based on my method of using subnuclear vacuoles, showed little difference between most of the progestogens as they are metabolised to norethisterone in the body. The exception is norgestrel which is about four to five times more powerful than norethisterone. But all of these are at least a thousand times more powerful, dose for dose, than natural progesterone according to Professor Spellacy's metabolic results (see page 209).

In the London Trials in the sixties we found that as little as 0.1mg of norgestrel plus 0.05mg ethinyl oestradiol was progestogenic and strong enough to prevent pregnancies although it had a high incidence of irregular bleeding, while we had several pregnancies with 1mg norethisterone acetate plus 0.05mg ethinyl oestradiol.

Some years later, in the early seventies, pills with that labelled dose (norethisterone acetate 1mg plus ethinyl oestradiol 0.05mg) appeared on the market. Dr Mears asked me why this latest pill, unlike its predecessor, now gave good cycle control and allowed very few incidental pregnancies. I had asked the same question of a manufacturer and learned that pill hormones were being micronised so that smaller doses were more efficiently absorbed by the gut. Now apparently, low doses had the same biological effect as previously achieved by higher doses. But the inescapable fact of life is that *any* dose which prevents pregnancy will produce a multitude of biochemical and cellular changes.

The RCGP study[16] has been widely misquoted as not showing an increase in breast cancer. In spite of losing 58 per cent of its pill users, and although most women stopped the pill within three years, the figures showed in 1981 a statistically significant increase in breast cancer among women aged thirty to thirty-four at diagnosis. There were twenty-two cases among users and five among controls aged twenty-five to thirty-four but that difference did not reach significance for the wider age range.

The data from the smaller Oxford/FPA study[17] is also compatible with an increased risk. The figures doubled for those who had used the pill for more than four years and when the interval from first use was longer than twelve years, but the numbers of women were too few to reach statistical significance. Dr Klim McPherson, Professor Vessey and others wrote to the *Lancet* on 17 December to say that they had now found an increased use of oral contraceptives before the first full-term pregnancy in breast cancer patients in thier matched control study. This brought the number of such studies up to six (*see* Chapter 1). Their previous data published two years earlier in 1982 had suggested that the pill had 'a non-significant protective effect' probably because only 9 per cent of the women had used the pill before their first pregnancy. When more cases were added the risk increased to three times for women who had taken the pill for over four years before their first baby.

In November 1985 the Atlanta Centers for Disease Control published their latest paper on breast cancer and the pill.[18] Although, unlike six other studies, they found no statistical relationship between pill use and breast cancer all the fifteen cases diagnosed in 20—24 year olds occurred among women who had taken the pill and over 86 per cent of the 25—39 year olds with breast cancer had taken the pill. An accompanying *Lancet* editorial discussed these inconsistencies and cited increases in breast cancer appearing fifteen years after radiation exposure in Hiroshima and Nagasaki[19] and 22 years after exposure to stilboestrol in pregnancy.[20] The editor warned that early pill use may take 10—20 years to show up excess cases of breast cancer.

I have always maintained that it is only the high drop out rate which prevents an epidemic of pill deaths. If women were forced to take the pill, the increase of life threatening conditions would be indisputable.

The Depo-Provera Inquiry

This inquiry was held in London in 1983. The Minister of Health, Mr Kenneth Clarke, had refused permission for this long-acting progestogen, known as DMPA, to be injected for contraceptive use, against the advice of the CSM. The manufacturers requested an inquiry in the hope that the minister's decision would be overruled. A women's group which opposed its use led by the writer Jill Rakusen, Marge Berer and Jean Robinson had painstakingly gathered together written evidence which, like me, they submitted to the inquiry. They were not, however, allowed to give oral evidence — only witnesses called by the manufacturers were interviewed — and the women protested about this by having their photos taken by the press with their mouths gagged by plaster.

Among the evidence given at the inquiry was the fact that out of 583 mentally retarded women who had received long-term DMPA, three had died from breast cancer, which is about twenty-five times the expected incidence in the general population. Their ages were thirty-two, thirty-three and forty. Even today, with an increase in breast cancer of 40 per cent over the past twenty years, the chance of a woman aged twenty-five to thirty-four developing the disease each year is fifteen per 100,000. In spite of this and a mass of other worrying evidence, however, permission was given that Depo-Provera could be used for long-term contraception in women 'in whom other contraceptives are contra-indicated or have caused unacceptable side effects'.[21]

Mostly, Depo-Provera has been used in Thailand, and a television film has shown Dr Suporn of the University Hospital treating a case of cervical cancer. She was anxious in case the increasing numbers were due to the pill or DMPA. Yet a leader in the *British Medical Journal* quoted this film as giving evidence that doctors in Thailand found the drug valuable.[22] Four studies though have found up to three times the risk of cervical cancer and even the inquiry concluded 'it seems likely that DMPA users constitute a relatively high risk group'.

Women's groups, including 'Ban the Jab', are most worried about the effects of this progestogen on the child during early pregnancy and lactation. A recent patient developed an unusual vascular cancer of the tongue when she was nine years old. Her mother had taken such a progestogen in pregnancy. A large Jerusalem study found a significant increase in vascular skin malformations in children whose mothers had taken the pill although there was a decreased risk if the mother had left a gap of one month before becoming pregnant after stopping the pill. In one study, 8 per cent of babies exposed to DMPA in early pregnancy had abnormalities at birth.[23]

Choriocarcinomas (malignant moles)

Women taking progestogen-only contraceptives run more risk of an ectopic pregnancy, especially if they already have diseased tubes due to infection. Hydatidiform moles can form if any products of conception remain in the womb or in a fallopian tube after a miscarriage or abortion. The combined pill trebles the risk of a mole changing into a highly invasive and vascular choriocarcinoma. These malignant tumours are never seen in animals but are becoming much more common since the widespread use of low dose pills has increased the unplanned pregnancy risk. The latest research by Professor Bagshawe and his team at Charing Cross Hospital is investigating whether the risk is even greater with a progestogen-only pill but the evidence suggests that it is especially dangerous to use progestogens for irregular bleeding after a pregnancy. I remember one of our first cases of choriocarcinoma in a pill taker was treated by Professor Bagshawe as early as 1963.

Sex Hormone Dependent Cancers

Before 1960 reproductive organ cancers were rare in young women and these cancers previously only increased in incidence after the menopause. Even today most reproductive cancers occur in older women.[24] Breast cancer is most common in the over eighties, while ovarian and endometrial cancers are likeliest in seventy-year-olds. While young women pill users need frequent cervical smears, the highest incidence or carcinoma of the cervix is in the age group sixty to seventy. Although the peak early cancer in situ incidence has shifted to the thirty to forty age group, it is still older women who are in the greatest need of lifesaving cervical screening. And yet there has been a great deal of publicity claiming that pill use prevents endometrial and ovarian cancer.

The American Walnut Creek study gives the best comparison so far published of the frequency of common cancers and pelvic disease.[25] Only the data for women pill users under the age of forty is useful, however, as because so many of the older 'control' women used oestrogens they had a very high incidence of breast, endometrial, ovarian and cervical

Walnut Creek

OC Use at Entry — Dec '68 to Feb '72

Never used OC

Age	Total women	Oestrogen Users (%)
18-39	2556	123 (4.8)
40-49	2664	623 (23.4)
50 +	1283	640 (49.9)

Ever used OC

Age	Total women	Oestrogen Users (%)
18-39	7506	359 (4.8)
40-49	2198	444 (20.2)
50 +	431	206 (47.8)

Figure 5

Walnut Creek

Follow-up to December 1977 — 86.2%
Number of women

Never used OC

Age	Pelvic Inflam. disease	Ovarian retention cysts	Adeno-myosis	Iron def. anaemia (acute)	Fibroma	Cervical cancer	Hysterectomy
18-39	7	4	3	1	20	1	63
40-49	9	11	16	16	82	5	239
50 +	8	10	36	10	55	6	222

Ever used OC

Age	Pelvic Inflam. disease	Ovarian retention cysts	Adeno-myosis	Iron def. anaemia (acute)	Fibroma	Cervical cancer	Hysterectomy
18-39	67*	50*	26*	25*	95*	37*	470*
40-49	26*	17	55*	12	195*	12	454*
50 +	4	6	38*	6	61*	0	177

*sign. past users.

Figure 6

Walnut Creek

Follow-up to December 1977 – 86.2%
Number of women with Malignant Neoplasms

Never used OC

Age	Breast	Endometrium	Ovary	Cervix
18-39	6	1	1	1
40-49	22	7*	6	5
50 +	36	32*	5	6

Ever used OC

Age	Breast	Endometrium	Ovary	Cervix
18-39	10	3	0	37*
40-49	36	4	3	12
50 +	21	11	1	0

*significant according to standardised rates.

Figure 7

Walnut Creek

Follow-up to December 1977 – 86.2%
Number of women with Malignant Neoplasms

Never used OC

Age	Melanoma	Others	Total
18-39	0	1	10
40-49	2	11	53
50 +	2	21	102

Ever used OC

Age	Melanoma	Others	Total
18-39	5*	9	64
40-49	7*	14	76
50 +	4*	14	51

*significant according to standardised rates.

Figure 8

cancers. Among these younger women the common cancers were: thirty-eight cervix, sixteen breast, four endometrial, one ovary, five melanoma, and ten others. Melanomas were significantly increased among pill users in all age groups a finding which may be related to the fact that the pill interferes with serotonin and melanin metabolism.

This means that reproductive cancers outnumbered all other cancers by four to one among these young women of whom 76 per cent had used hormones. In the 1930s one in seven of the population died of cancer but in the 1980s one in five is dying. In women of all ages one third of cancers were hormone related before the pill.

Endometrial Cancer

In the Walnut Creek study there were three oral contraceptive endometrial cancers to one control aged under forty. Among the over fifties there were eleven cancers among pill users to thirty-three among controls, but among the women over fifty there were three times more control women and three times more of them had used oestrogens. It is admitted that oestrogen use significantly increases the risk of endometrial cancer — a fact which is no longer in doubt. So much so that many women are advised to have hysterectomies before having 'hormone replacement treatment' to remove their risk of endometrial or cervical cancer. But the Walnut Creek study also shows a significant increase in pelvic diseases and reports a huge number of hysterectomies carried out among the under forties and forty- to fifty-year-olds who used the pill. They were more likely to get pelvic inflammatory disease, fibroids and adenomyosis — gland tissue in the womb muscle.

If more pill users have hysterectomies, a case control study of women with endometrial cancer could give the impression that the pill prevents endometrial cancer. And this is what has happened. Dr Howard Ory of the US Centers for Disease Control in Atlanta, Georgia, is among those who have

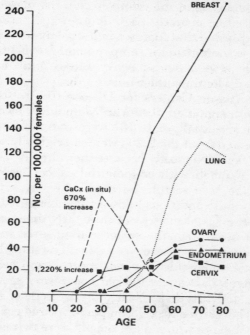

Cancer registrations per 100,000 females 1981
(increase since registration started 1962)

Figure 9

published the evidence that women with endometrial and ovarian cancer are less likely to have ever used the pill and because of this and similar results has suggested that pill use prevents large numbers of women being sent to hospital for benign breast disease, endometrial and ovarian cancer, ovarian retention cysts, ectopic pregnancies, pelvic inflammatory disease, iron-deficiency anaemia and rheumatoid arthritis.[26] But the Walnut Creek study found significant increases in most of these conditions either among ever users at entry or later in the trial. It even had more young pill users

133

admitted to hospital for severe iron deficiency anaemia due to heavy periods. Although progestogen pills dry up and atrophy the lining of the womb so that the usual pill withdrawal bleeding is much less than a normal period, I have already explained that some women still have overdeveloped arterioles in their atrophic samples and I frequently found I could only stop irregular heavy bleeding by asking the women to discontinue their pills.

In the Atlanta Centers for Disease Control study, 262 women with endometrial cancer[27] were interviewed by telephone but eventually only 187 were compared with 1,320 controls taken from the 2,208 women originally selected — 553 were excluded mostly because they already had a hysterectomy. Women with endometrial cancer were twice as likely to be overweight, infertile, have hypertension or diabetes — all conditions known to be increased by pill or hormone use. Cancer cases were also three times less likely to have ever been pregnant for more than seven months and twice as likely to have used oestrogens. The study had half as many cases under thirty-four as controls and most women with endometrial cancer (69 per cent) were aged between forty-five and fifty-five. Nearly 60 per cent of the cancer cases had never used the pill compared with 44 per cent of the controls. Women who did use the pill were twice as likely to stop within one year. These same facts have been interpreted as further proof that 'pill use prevents' with the risk 'reduced from 1 to 0.5' — cut by half.

The fact that fewer cases ever took the pill does not necessarily mean that it is protective when taken. This point was picked up by Professor Philip Burch, an expert in medical physics, who wrote to the *Lancet* saying that such negative associations did not prove protection and that to claim so was a misuse of statistics and showed an inadequacy of logic.

Ovarian Cancer

The same sort of arguments apply to this story. Again, the incidence in young women is very low but the position in older women is confused by oestrogen use — and by the use of talcum powder.

As part of my Family Planning training I was told that rubber diaphragms and cervical caps should be kept dry when not in use by a liberal dusting of talcum powder. In the mid-seventies it became common knowledge that talcum in the pelvis could cause ovarian cancer just as asbestos particles can cause lung cancer. Since then talcum use has been discouraged as studies showed that cap users had double the risk of ovarian cancer.[28] Like testicular cancer in men, ovarian cancer is also more likely to develop in women with congenital abnormalities of their sex organs, possibly due to hormone influences before or at birth.

Several epidemiological studies also suggest that pill use reduces the risk of ovarian cancer, again because fewer cases overall took the pill. One of these studies[29] from the Atlanta Centers for Disease Control recorded 237 cases of ovarian cancer and enrolled 179 of these women aged twenty to fifty-four. This time, of the 2,208 normal women initially selected as controls, 1,642 were used, and 226 women with no ovaries at the time of the telephone interview were excluded. Once more, women with cancer were twice as likely to be infertile, and half as likely to have ever married or had children. Although the chance of an average women developing ovarian cancer when she is between the ages of twenty and twenty-nine is only two per 100,000 per year, in this study 15.1 per cent of the cancers were in this group. Most women under forty (80—90 per cent) had used the pill but most of the cases (68 per cent) were over forty. No details of oestrogen use were given. The cancer women who had taken the pill were more likely to have given it up within their first two years of use and more likely to have done so recently within the preceding ten years.

The claim that the results of such studies can be used to 'estimate that more than 1,700 cases of ovarian cancer are averted each year by past or current oral contraceptive use among women in the United States' does not, in my opinion, inevitably follow.

The argument is that the pill stops ovulation and non-functioning ovaries are less likely to develop cysts or become malignant but two-thirds of new cases of ovarian cancer occur in women between the ages of fifty-five and eighty whose ovaries have long ceased to function.

The Walnut Creek trial also found that if women they had enrolled had ever used the pill they had significantly more ovarian cysts and at their ten-year follow up fifty younger pill users had retention cysts compared with four in the control group. This effect had been predicted by the discoverer of stilboestrol — Professor Sir Charles Dodds.

The weight of evidence, especially when animal and biochemical studies are taken into account, is that hormone use is likely to increase the risk of ovarian disease and malignancies. Again, the fact that large numbers of women have ovariectomies as well as hysterectomies may be preventing a rise in ovarian cancer incidence over all.

Fortunately, new methods of screening can show up ovarian disease at an early stage and should prevent an increase in ovarian cancer morality which would seem inevitable among females exposed to hormones at early stages of foetal development.

Dr Regina Schoental of the Royal Veterinary College has emphasised that exposure to oestrogenic substances is the main cause of reproductive cancers.[30] Oestrogens occur naturally in plants in the form of mycotoxins. Fungicides prevent infestation with mycotoxins but too little simply encourages their production. They accumulate in mouldy grains and in animal fatty tissues. They are present especially in cereals, eggs; milk and beer.

Countries like Ireland, Scotland and Scandinavia, with cold, wet climates, had a high incidence of breast cancer before the pill as damp conditions increase the levels of naturally occurring oestrogenic substances. As the natural background level of oestrogen intake is anyway high, Dr Schoental is completely against adding oestrogens in the form of the pill or hormone treatments as they can be the final straw that breaks the camel's back.[31]

There is a great deal of difference between a good doctor and a bad doctor but very little difference between a good doctor and no doctor at all.

This piece of wisdom, penned by Benjamin Franklin in 1787, is the perfect motto for our Clinical Ecology Society, and in 1977 Dr Ralph Paffenbarger referred to it in his paper on breast cancer[32] when he said: 'These potent contraceptive drugs, available on prescription, incite considerable metabolic activity and are known to be carcinogenic in animal experiments. In writing these prescriptions, we physicians must ask ourselves if Franklin would be classifying us as good or bad doctors.'

Dr Theron Randolph founded modern clinical ecology after seeing the disastrous effects of steroids such as cortisone and predisone on the future health of his patients. He believes, as I do, that no one should lightly be given long-term steroids, and that includes the euphemistically termed pill. Dr Beaumont's team in Paris have provided us with an immunological basis for Randolph's observation — Beaumont talks of two months on the pill causing years of immunological scarring with altered anti-body levels to several steroids.[33] Dr Ifor Capel and his team from the Marie Curie Memorial laboratories found fundamental changes in the red cells of girls taking low dose pills by seven months of them starting. The changes in glutathione peroxidase levels are even greater than in older women with breast cancer.[34] He thinks there is a reversal of the normal anti-oxidant mechanisms which are essential for the healthy reproduction of our cells. The pill-caused changes in liver also mean that mutagens and carcinogens will be less easily detoxified during or after pill use.

It is against this background of biochemical and immune changes that we have to consider the dramatic rise in cancer in young women in the last twenty years. Breast cancer incidence has increased by 40 per cent in England and Wales and the death rate by 25 per cent. Papers from Paffenbarger, Fasal, Pike, Jick and others have all found significant

137

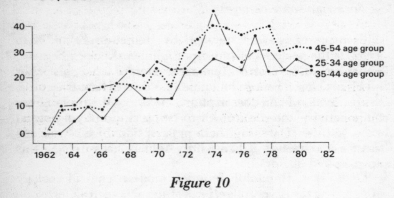

Breast cancer % increase in registrations per 100,000 females

Figure 10

increases in the incidence of breast cancer in women which multiply with duration of pill use, younger age at first starting the pill and previous benign breast disease — especially if the breast disease started when they were given hormones, or if a mother or sister has had breast cancer. Unlike the 'pill prevents' papers which claim pill use reduces the cancer risk by half, the recriminating research finds increases are much larger. Dr Elfriede Fasal found the few who had used the pill for over six years, and had a history of benign breast disease, had an eleven times increased risk.[35]

Dr Hershel Jick found in her case control study that older pre-menopausal women aged forty-six to fifty with breast cancer were four times more likely to be taking the pill and women between fifty-one and fifty-five were about 15.5 times more likely to be recent or current users.[36]

In 1970 MacMahon showed that women who have a first child before the age of twenty have half the risk of developing breast cancer while first time mothers over thirty-five have twice the risk.[37] The obstetrician James Owen Drife and his

138

colleagues more recently found that it is only after a first full-term pregnancy that the breast tissue starts to respond to cyclic progesterone. An early abortion may increase the risk. Until the first child, a woman's breast tissue is not prepared for breast feeding and is unresponsive to progesterone. The glands only react to oestrogens and seem more likely to be overstimulated into cancerous overgrowth. So Drife theorises that if a young woman taking the pill has immature breast tissue which does not respond to the progestogen component she is more at risk from the unopposed oestrogen in the pill. Mr Drife said if the pill did double the risk of breast cancer this would be very serious because it is so common.[38]

America's Devastated Women?

In July 1984 a large case control study from Boston, Philadelphia and New York, was published in *JAMA (The Journal of the American Medical Association)*.[39] It was hailed as being the latest proof that oestrogens did not cause breast cancer. 1,610 women with breast cancer, average age fifty-one, were compared with a control group of hospital patients with the same average age. All the women were carefully questioned and their memories jogged to make sure non-contraceptive use of oestrogens for a multitude of 'gynaecological' conditions was not overlooked. The control group started as 6,017 women, average age thirty-nine, but 1,606 women were randomly picked out to age match the smaller number with breast cancer. The controls had never had cancer and were in hospital because of trauma, disc disorders, digestive disorders, acute infections and various other conditions.

'Despite the lack of biologic plausibility' women who had had their ovaries removed before the menopause appeared to have less risk of breast cancer if they had used conjugated oestrogens in the distant past. When we take a closer look at this extraordinary paper we notice that 70 per cent of the controls and 57 per cent of the breast cancer cases had reached the menopause — but one in three controls did so before the age of forty, compared with one in eight cases. Nearly half of the women with breast cancer reached the menopause at the normal age of fifty or more but only a quarter of the control women did so. Seven out of ten control women who used conjugated oestrogens for at least five years had their menopause caused by surgical removal of their womb or both ovaries.

Whereas some control women in the Walnut Creek oral contraceptive study had used oestrogens, this study goes a step further. There is no mention of oral contraceptive use at all. Considering the Walnut Creek study found highly significant increases with pill use in ovarian disease, uterine disease and hysterectomies in women under forty — very few of whom had used oestrogens — it seems most unlikely that 6,017 hospital patients, average age thirty-nine, in America between 1976 and 1981 had never taken oestrogens and progestogens in the form of oral contraceptives. The claim that women with breast cancer tend to have a late menopause may derive from the fact that other women with ovary or womb disorders tend to have an unnaturally early menopause because of surgical intervention.

DES

In 1938 Professor Sir Charles Dodds and his colleagues discovered that a non-steroid compound, diethyl stilboestrol (DES) acted like an oestrogen. It does not have the complete four ring steroid structure of oestrogen and progestogens but its molecules are arranged in such a way that it has the same key groupings. It locks into the oestrogen receptors in our cells so exactly that the cell is fooled into thinking the body's own oestrogens are telling it to act in a certain way such as growing rapidly and dividing.

After a baby is born the breast responds to the brain hormone prolactin and secretes milk. The more the baby sucks, the more milk is produced until the correct amount is being supplied for the baby's needs. It is precisely at this critical and important time that doctors began to give oestrogens to mothers who did not want to nurse their babies. Oestrogens can, via a feedback mechanism, switch off the prolactin and stop milk production. If a mother was making too much milk, oestrogens — mostly stilboestrol — were also given to treat 'breast engorgement'. Stilboestrol was available on a large scale from 1941 and was widely used until the 1970s. In 1967 my senior lecturer in Dundee, now Professor Alex Turnbull in Oxford, and his colleagues discovered that many of the women having thrombosis after childbirth were taking oestrogens. In fact, women given oestrogens were three times more likely to develop clots than other new mothers.[40]

Hospital doctors stopped giving oestrogens to lactating women. If the baby does not suckle the milk production dried up automatically so nature achieves the same result spontaneously without resorting to drugs. Only a few doctors still prescribe oestrogens for lactating women, and sometimes women have to be sent to hospital because they have withdrawal bleeding a day or two after taking these unnecessary hormones.

Our breast cancer rates really began to increase in the 1960s, but oestrogens had already started to be used in a number of ways. In 1947 the US government allowed stilboestrol to be used for the 'caponisation' of poultry. Since then a variety of sex hormones have been given to poultry, beef, pigs and even sheep. Oestrogens, progesterone, progestogens and testosterone have been injected or implanted into animals to promote growth and feed efficiency. The animals become heavy, mostly because of fluid retention, even if they eat less.

Just as prescribing the contraceptive pill has been an easy source of income for many of the world's doctors, injecting hormones into animal livestock has become an important part of a veterinary surgeon's routine. The advertising blurbs sent to farmers assures of efficiency, safety and lack of harmful effects in spite of the wealth of research findings to the contrary. Oestrogens, progestogens and androgens have caused cancer in humans, mice, rats, dogs and monkeys. Oestrogens have caused cancer of the breast, endometrium, cervix, vagina, ovary, testes, pituitary, kidney, bladder, adrenals, liver and lymphoid tissue. Progesterone and progestogens have caused cancer of the breast, endometrium, cervix, ovary, pituitary and liver. Androgens have caused liver and uterine cancer.[41]

Before powerful hormones were so widely dispensed in this indiscriminate fashion, cancer was mostly a disease of old age. As we grow older our enzymes and homeostatic mechanisms become less able to cope. Our cells need continual renewal and as we age we are less able to do this effectively. Bad eating and drinking habits and toxic chemicals in our environment begin to take their toll. Our chances of developing most types of cancer used to increase after the age of fifty, but soon this may be no longer the case. During the last few decades the increase in cancer has been greatest among young adults.

It is usually people in the lower social classes who are most likely to suffer illness. They may be short of nutritious food and, in industrial societies, they are also more likely to live near dense traffic fumes or be subject to toxic chemicals at work. It is the well off, however, the doctors, managers and teachers who are most likely to develop testicular cancer between ages twenty-five and thirty-five,[42] and it is women in social class 1 who are most likely to get breast cancer.

So why are the young and the well-off the prime targets of our present cancer epidemic? Is it because higher social class women were the first to try the new oral contraceptive pills, more likely to take hormones during pregnancy to prevent miscarriage and more likely to take 'replacement' oestrogens for menopausal symptoms? I believe it is. I think women have been unnecessarily taking hormones over the past decades. The rise in cervical cancer following the rise in sexually transmitted diseases in the two world wars had an observed latent period of twenty years. But it is a cause for great concern that young women are showing an immediate rise in cancer incidence long before twenty years of oral contraceptive use. Young women are now getting rapidly progressive cancers well before the age when cancer is more likely, and the numbers are projected to increase.

How many of us can say we have been good doctors?

The Effect of Hormones on Older Women

Although only about two per cent of British women have taken hormones at the menopause, as many as fifty per cent of women attending many American centres have been given hormone replacement therapy (HRT). Many are young women in their 30s and 40s who have used the pill and had surgical removal of their womb or ovaries. In Britain there is now an advertising campaign aimed at persuading more women to take hormones. Most women find their periods become less frequent and stop finally between 50 and 52. Smokers tend to have their menopause at younger ages. Although fertility declines sharply with age a woman is still capable of becoming pregnant for up to two years after her last period. As the ovaries stop producing large amounts of oestrogens and progesterone common symptoms are flushing, sweating, vaginal dryness and sudden ageing. Naturally women are keen to prevent these distressing problems.

In an article in the *British Medical Journal*[43] benefits of hormone therapy listed include:
Curing flushing and sweating
Preventing vaginal dryness
Preventing osteoporosis
Curing or preventing ageing changes in the vagina and urethra.

143

Disadvantages listed are:

Continuing to have periods and the increased risk of endometrial cancer. Samples are taken every two years

Unknown long term risks of breast cancer and heart disease

Dependency on oestrogens, that is, severe withdrawal symptoms

Progestogens are now added to oestrogens hopefully to diminish the risk of endometrial cancer. The progestogen only pills now being recommended for women over 35 can cause irregular bleeding and menstrual chaos.

Osteoporosis (thinning of the bones)

Thin bones which break easily are a common problem for eighty year old women. For some of them the slightest trauma can mean a broken forearm, hip or even a vertebra.

Our bones become thinner as we grow older but if we have eaten a good diet since childhood with plenty of first class protein, calcium and Vitamin D, and if we take lots of exercise and avoid excessive stress smoking or drinking alcohol, we are unlikely to suffer from serious osteoporosis, at least until we are in our eighties. However, auto-immune disease has increased far more in women than men, and such patients are likely to be given steroids like prednisone. But using steroids increases the chance of fractures by about nine times. No wonder the numbers of old people with osteoporosis has rocketed.

There is concern in industrialised societies that toxic metals, lead from traffice fumes, cadmium from cigarettes, aluminium from the packaging of convenience foods, and mercury from tooth fillings, may be interfering with bone metabolism. We have recently found that children with zinc deficiency have not only very small amounts of zinc in their sweat but they also have significantly more lead and cadmium compared with children who have normal

144

amounts of sweat zinc, lead and cadmium concentrate in the bones displacing calcium.

The daily requirement of calcium officially recommended in the UK is only 500 mg and often daily intakes are lower than this, especially among individuals who avoid cow's milk because of allergy problems. Balance studies have shown that women need 1100mg of calcium each day but after the menopause they need more — 1500mg daily. One study found women with osteoporosis had low milk consumption, poor lactose absorption and flat glucose tolerance curves.[44]

A *Lancet* editorial in June 1985 said there was now sufficient evidence that a boost of calcium intake might favourably affect bone mass and, unlike other approaches to osteoporosis (such as hormone replacement therapy), this strategy would be free from toxic side effects.[45]

Special tests have shown that women taking oestrogens after their natural or surgically induced menopause do not lose their bone tissue so quickly. But as usual very little is said about the huge drop out rates and about the reasons most women stop taking these hormones within two or three years.

The sudden fall in ovarian oestrogens and progesterone and rise in corticosteriods at the menopause mean women start to lose their bone tissue more quickly than men but 20 per cent of women do so more rapidly than the remainder of the population. Women who have abnormal adrenal function, perhaps due to long term use of the pill, would be especially susceptible to early osteoporosis because the adrenals normally boost oestrogen production at the menopause.

Women have a lower risk of heart attacks than men until fourteen years after the menopause. Whatever the age of the menopause, whether 35 or 55, whether it has been natural or surgically induced, women begin to develop atherosclerosis about fourteen years later when they catch up with the male pattern of high risk. Pill deaths in young women are not usually due to atherosclerosis but to the other vascular changes I have already described.

Because oestrogens raise the protective fraction of cholesterol optimistic gynaecologists hope that oestrogens, given to treat menopausal symptoms or to prevent long term osteoporosis, will actually prevent heart disease. This betrays an amazingly simplistic approach and a dismissal of all the many vascular changes and metabolic upsets such as low zinc, high copper and raised cortiocosteroids induced by oestrogens.

Although as many as a third or a half of newly postmenopausal women have been given 'replacement' oestrogens at some American centres of excellence very few women over 60 still take them.

In October 1985 the prestigious *New England Journal of Medicine* published two papers. One, from Harvard, gave results supporting the hypothesis that post menopausal use of oestrogen reduced the risk of severe coronary disease.[46] The other paper from the Framingham Heart Study group reported that their post menopausal oestrogen users had 50 per cent more cardiovascular and twice as much cerebrovascular disease as non-users.[47] How can there be such different results?

In the Framingham study older women, aged between 50 and 83, were examined carefully and their electrocardiogram readings were checked. At the last examination about 17 per cent of the women in their 50s but only 2 per cent of those over 70 were still taking hormones. 60 per cent had taken oestrogens for three years. Oestrogen users' higher risk of vascular disease was independent of other main known risks such as early menopause. While oestrogen users weighed less and had lower risk cholesterol profiles than the control women, they also had had these advantages *before* they started taking oestrogens. In other words, *lower risk women are selected for oestrogen hormone replacement therapy*. Women selected may either have no obvious side effects on the pill, or if they did have problems they might be unaware of that these have been caused or exacerbated by the pill. Although nearly a third of the oestrogen users had had a surgical menopause (and the Walnut Creek data showed significant increases in hysterectomies, pelvic and ovarian disease among young pill users) the women likely to get pelvic disease may not be the ones who are most susceptible to vascular disease.

In the Harvard study younger women (nurses aged between 30 and 55) were surveyed by post over a period of six years at two yearly intervals. Women taking oestrogens were five times more likely to have lost their ovaries but they were nearly twice as likely to have taken the pill. At each survey, as women who had already got coronary disease might 'alter their pattern of hormone use' (that is, stop taking oestrogens) and, as they were at 'increased risk to progression of the disease' they were excluded from further follow up. There was no reduction in total mortality once 'women with cancer at base line were eliminated'. The proportion of deaths due to confirmed coronary disease was small. The paper concluded the beneficial effects on osteoporosis or menopausal symptoms had to be weighed against the the well-recognised increase in endometrial cancer and possibly breast cancer.

Is it sacrilege to suggest that the pill may be actually causing osteoporosis? Dr Kitty Little is in no doubt. She says alternating high levels of oestrogen with stress (high adrenal cortocoid hormones) is the most effective way of removing bone tissue. Also, oestrogens and progestogens (now added to 'replacement' oestrogens to lessen the womb cancer risk) are strongly thrombogenic — that is likely to cause small clots (microthrombi) in the bones. And yet these possibilities are receiving little study, interest or follow up in the large pill studies.[48] Women taking the pill have lower than normal levels of oestrogen and low oestrogen can cause osteoporosis. We found that progestogens decreased alkaline phosphatase activity in the endometrium and progestogens, while preventing bone breakdown, actually reduced bone formation as judged by blood enzyme levels. Sleby and Peacock from an MRC mineral unit in Leeds found that oestrogen reduces

147

bone formation and adding progestogen further depresses it.

There are reports of osteoporosis in teenagers with anorexia.[49] This low zinc state probably involves many deficiencies including interference with bone metabolism. Osteoporosis in pregnancy with low plasma vitamin D levels has been described as a failure of the maternal skeleton to prepare for the stress of childbirth.[50] Women taking oestrogens have changes showing that they are already under abnormal stress. They do not have the increases in prolactin, the lactation hormone in response to stress because their levels are too high already due to their abnormally high copper levels.[51] This high prolactin is suggested as a reason women taking oestrogens are more likely to get pituitary tumours which secrete prolactin (prolactinomas) and more likely to get breast cancer. As anti-oestrogen therapy is now being promoted as treatment for breast cancer why are women still being given oestrogens for frivolous reasons such as preventing wrinkles or flushing?

Mrs SE came to see me with an anxiety state and a diagnosis of Sjögren's syndrome. She was 51 and had been taking oestrogens since she was 38 following a hysterectomy for fibroids. One ovary was removed and the other was shrivelled, she was told. She didn't take hormones for a year but her vagina felt dry so she was given oestrogens. At first she felt normal and happy but she then developed arthritis and back pain. Gradually her eyes and throat felt more dried up, especially when she ate cakes or drank alcohol. Sjögren's syndrome was diagnosed (an autoimmune condition which can be a reaction to drugs). She was told to increase her dose of oestrogen. She had a frightening attack of chest pain and a friend who had recently stopped taking oestrogens herself because of a deep vein thrombosis suggested Mrs SE contact me. Her mineral analysis showed very low zinc in her blood, sweat and hair. She also had high toxic metals in her hair with mercury especially elevated. Stopping oestrogens, a low allergy diet and supplements of minerals, vitamins and essential oils resulted in immediate improvement. She had a strong allergy to yeast, the likely cause of the problems in the first place.

For decades oestrogens have been sold to women as the secret of eternal youth. As ovarian, endometrial, cervical and breast cancers are still increasing it is hard to come to any other conclusion than that the main beneficiaries of oestrogen treatment are the drug companies.

Summary

Pill induced overgrowth or atrophy of the target sex organs increases the risk of cancer. Pill induced vascularity increases the risk of spread.

Cervical cancer

* Risk of early cervical cancer was less than 1 in 100,000 in 1965

* First reports of large increases due to the pill in 1968

* By 1980 1 in 25 women had a positive smear at a London Family Planning clinic

* Invasive cancers are increasingly fatal in under 40s

Breast cancer

* Breast cancer is very rare under age 25 but the numbers doubled in the 70s compared with the 60s

* Longer pill use before first baby increases later risk

* In 1982 breast cancer was the commonest single cause of death in women aged between 25 and 44 — 836 deaths compared with 235 due to road accidents

* Women taking the pill in their early 50s may have more than 15 times increased risk of breast cancer

Ovarian cancer

* Ovarian cancer is very rare in women under 44 with only 411 new cases in 1981, but in the same year 6,500 women under 44 had their diseased ovaries removed surgically

* Eighty per cent of women developing ovarian cancer under 40 are known to have taken the pill

* There is therefore no real evidence that pill use prevents ovarian cancer in young women

Endometrial cancer

* Endometrial cancer is extremely rare in women under 44 with only 119 new cases in 1981, but in the same year 34,590 women under 44 had their wombs removed surgically

* Seventy-five per cent of women developing endometrial cancer under 40 are known to have taken the pill

* Again there is therefore no real evidence that pill use prevents endometrial cancer in young women

Osteoporosis

* How does the pill cause osteoporosis?
  * Abnormally high corticosteriods (stress response)
  * Multiple microthrombi in bones
  * Altered alkaline phosphatase activity

* *Zinc deficiency*

  • Malabsorption — especially affecting milk and calcium
  • candida
  • food allergies
  • accumulation of toxic metals in bones

* *High copper*

  Liver dysfunction and interference with calcium and vitamin D metabolism

* Reduces bone formation — especially important in teenagers.

8 What is Happening to the Young?

Common belief: *Hormones only affect a fetus if they are taken during pregnancy.*

Fact: *Pill use can make a woman unfit for pregnancy.*

Cancer in Children

In 1971 the bombshell burst. Dr Arthur Herbst and his colleagues at the Massachusetts General Hospital in Boston proved beyond doubt that exposure to oestrogens (DES) in pregnancy had caused cancer of the vagina in teenage girls.

The fact that exposure to hormones in early fetal life or at birth can lead to life-long consequences might never have become general knowledge if the tumour had been a common one like carcinoma in situ of the cervix. Instead, the clear cell adenocarcinoma of the vagina is so unusual that between 1966 and publication in 1971[1] Dr Herbst diagnosed far more cases than had ever been discovered before. A search of the entire medical literature yielded only four reports in women under thirty years of age.

Why was this rare tumour becoming common in the Boston area? A fashion had begun in the late 1940s[2] to give stilboestrol to 'prevent miscarriages' in habitual aborters. Its chief proponent, Dr George Smith, head of Harvard's gynaecology department and his wife Olive advised its use to make 'abnormal pregnancy more normal'. From Boston the use of DES spread and by the 1950s it was being widely prescribed throughout the USA and, although less frequently, in many other countries. It is estimated that nearly two million women in the USA were given the drug and 7,800 in the UK.[3] These are probably underestimates as some obstetricians declined to co-operate in making their records available to the investigators. The doses had ranged from 1.5 to 225mg daily over periods varying from one week to the entire length of pregnancy.

In 1953 a study from Chicago, reported in the *American Journal of Obstetrics and Gynecology*,[4] failed to substantiate any demonstrable therapeutic effect on preventing miscarriage, and in fact there were indications that hormone therapy increased the risks of bleeding. After this the treatment began to fall out of fashion. Once the link had been made between the tumour and the mother's oestrogen use, national registers were set up and the exposed population has since been kept under close scrutiny.

By 1981, 400 cases of the once rare adenocarcinoma had been recorded. Follow-up of these cases showed that the cancer could be extremely virulent, with rapid spread to other regions of the body. Death had occurred in over a quarter and recurrences after surgery had been frequent in those who had survived. These 400 cases were only a small proportion of those affected.

Non-malignant tissue changes were present in over 60 per cent of all women known to have been exposed to DES in early fetal life. The most common finding was areas of glandular tissue (adenosis) in the vagina. As in cases with overt cancer such tissue had been found near or around the tumours, it was feared to be a pre-cancerous lesion. The DES daughters have been regularly inspected and adenosis is surgically excised when it is found. But other more common female genital tract cancers such as carcinoma in situ have also been found more frequently in this population.

So far there has only been one case described in the British literature. In 1979 my pathologist friend Dr John

Pryse-Davies and his colleagues described their findings. A woman who had been exposed to stilboestrol in utero had extensive adenosis of her cervix and vagina at the age of twenty-three. Four years later she developed a grade III cervical carcinoma in situ after taking oral contraceptives.[5]

How much of our present epidemic of cervical cancer is due to exposure to hormones in utero or at birth? Just as the lining of the cervix in teenagers is changing from an immature cell type to an adult type and is especially sensitive to exogenous hormones, the developing cervix in a fetus is also particularly vulnerable to hormone influences. Animal studies have clearly shown that exposure to hormones, especially in early fetal life or at birth, can affect cell memory. These cells become particularly sensitive to either exogenous hormones like the pill or even rising levels of endogenous natural hormones at puberty. Not only were oestrogens given to suppress lactation, or progestogens given as contraceptives to lactating mothers, but some obstetricians even gave large doses of oestrogens to induce labour.

Labour is induced by pituitary hormones — pitocin or oxytocin and now by prostaglandins. It is a cause for great concern that adequate life studies are not always carried out in animals, and when they are, are ignored or regarded as irrelevant, which happened with the pill. There are remarkably few follow-up studies carried out on children but the evidence of increasing mental handicap, hyperactivity, dyslexia and behavioural problems suggest that such work is of the highest priority. Within two or three years the effects on several generations of animals can be witnessed. Dr Schoental has carried out invaluable work showing the effect of oestrogenic substances on the offspring of rats. These animals rarely attack mice but after fetal exposure to oestrogens they will kill a mouse placed in their cage. Besides changes in behaviour, the rats have more abnormalities of their sex organs and are more likely to develop tumours.[6]

It has been recorded that there are now seven times more boys being born with an undescended testicle than there were in 1969.[7a] As many as one in ten boys are affected and one in thirty-three are operated on before they are two years old to reduce their risk of infertility and testicular cancer. The numbers of these operations in boys up to age four years has increased ten times between 1962 and 1981.

The incidence of testicular cancer has also increased among young men in the past twenty years. Oestrogen exposure increases the risk eight times,[7b] but the use of progesterone, progestogens or the pill in pregnancy may also have countributed to the increase over the last 40 years.

A letter to the *Lancet* in February 1984[8] described how when men took MPA tablets and applied testosterone ointment to their skin each day as a contraceptive, their female partners had raised levels of testosterone and began to grow hair on their upper lips and thighs. This begs a question. Does a man having sexual intercourse with a woman on the pill run an increased risk of testicular cancer either due to absorbing the progestogens, which have male hormone-like actions, or by developing antibodies to them?

Dr Schoental is extremely worried that test-tube babies are being exposed to hormones, and she believes such experiments should be stopped or halted until life experiments have been carried out on animals. It should be possible to predict the effects on the fetus when it is being manipulated at such a sensitive stage. Already babies have been born with obvious malformation after exposure to MPA, which is already used to aid implantation for test tube babies.

The full implications for the future of the children may not become clear in humans for as long as sixty years, but profit and expediency seem of more importance than the long-term human consequences.

Much of our infertility epidemic can be attributed to

taking the pill or using IUDs. IUDs increase the likelihood of tubal infections and permanent blockage. Pill taking increases the risk of infection also but many women are unable to ovulate after stopping the pill. They take hormones to block their biological clock and sometimes they can't start it again. It is young girls who have already shown a sensitivity to hormones who are more likely to be affected. If given the pill for irregular periods they have a 7.7 times increased risk of developing a pituitary prolactinoma tumour compared with women given the pill for contraception.[9]

The close scrutiny of the DES daughters has revealed that they have an increased incidence of miscarriage, ectopic pregnancy, stillbirth, premature labour and sterility.

Homosexuality

The DES sons have not escaped either. Besides having a high incidence of genital tract malformations, semen abnormalities, sterility, infertility and cancer of the testes, they are half as likely to marry as unexposed men of the same age.[3]

Masculinisation of female fetuses and feminisation of male fetuses have been demonstrated in animals experimentally exposed to hormones. Inevitably the question has arisen as to whether sexual orientation towards members of the same sex can be caused by exposure to sex hormones in utero or at birth and whether the recent apparent rise in homosexuality is entirely coincidental. A double blind study of MPA exposure showed the boys to be less aggressive and less interested in boy's toys. Girls became more tomboyish and were less interested in dolls.

There is a difference in amine balance and brain control in males and females. In animals it is known that one sex has more adrenaline control while the other has more serotonin control, and this can be switched by early hormone exposure. It is an interesting speculation that certain food preferences may be inborn — I am reminded that, as a general rule, men seem to prefer cheese whereas women prefer chocolate.

Foresight

There has been a tendency to say 'let's forget the DES story'. As it was specific to stilboestrol it can be abandoned as a lesson, but oestrogens act like oestrogens however they are made. In Britain we were fortunate that stilboestrol was used so little in pregnancy and we can thank Professor Sir Charles Dodds who, having developed the hormone was so against its use.

When I began to prescribe the pill he was president of the Royal College of Physicians and he strongly protested about the pill being given for contraception. He was well aware from his lifetime studies that all prescriptions of hormones could have dire results. He wrote: 'It is unlikely that one could submit the delicately balanced hormonal system of a woman to such violent alteration for forty years without something seriously happening.'[10]

Of course, we know that the average woman gives up the pill within a few years but exposure to extra hormones for one day only may be critical in the life of a child. The key times are very early in pregnancy, often before a woman even knows she is pregnant, and at birth.

Many charities and women's groups have been started to help deal with our present day epidemics of ill health. One of the most important of these in my opinion is 'Foresight'. This is the Association for the Promotion of Pre-Conceptual Care, which was the brainchild of Mrs Belinda Barnes and became a charity in 1978.

Mrs Barnes, as a nursery nurse and mother of three children, became acutely aware of the importance of correct infant feeding for the developing child. She met Dr

Elizabeth Lodge Rees, a Californian paediatrician who specialised in nutrition, allergies and hair mineral analysis.[11] For ten years Mrs Barnes has sent hair samples to be analysed by Dr Lodge Rees who has more than twenty years' experience of treating problem children using mineral analysis. Estimation of essential elements such as zinc, magnesium, manganese and chromium, and toxic metals such as lead, cadmium, mercury and aluminium in parts per million, is one of the most rapidly advancing areas in medicine in the eighties. Dr Lodge Rees was one of the first in this field and was the director of a mineral laboratory in California. She soon discovered that problem or sick children were likely to have deficiencies of nutritional elements and excesses of toxic elements. She developed treatments of vitamin and mineral supplementation and simple replacement methods for removing the toxic metals while continuing to monitor the results by repeated hair tests.

I first met both these outstanding ladies at a Foresight conference in 1978 at Charing Cross Hospital. Since then Mrs Barnes has invited me to lecture at many of her frequent Foresight conferences and teach-ins throughout the country. She also inspired me to review the literature on causes of congenital abnormalities[12] and come up with the term 'common social poisons', which means the pill, smoking, alcohol, drugs and unnecessary medications like tranquillisers.

The Foresight booklet, *Guidelines for Future Parents*[13], begins: 'Many people may wonder why pre-conceptual preparation is felt to be necessary. It may be felt that since time immemorial babies have been coming into the world with very little fuss and therefore why should it now be necessary to go to these lengths? Surely mankind is better housed, fed and cared for now than at any time in history?'

The most recent records show 3,631 stillborn (1983) 13,972 congenital abnormalities (1983) and 6,582 perinatal deaths (1983).

The 1983 notification rate for congenital abnormalities of

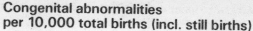

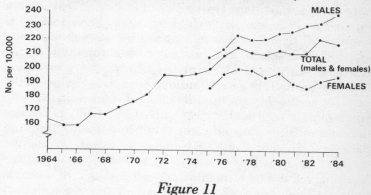

Figure 11

220.8 per 10,000 births is the highest since 1964, when registrations began to be published.

The Foresight Association believes that most of these
problems can be avoided with sufficient care and the
preparation of both parents before conception.

Dyslexia and Zinc Deficiency

Because of my own family history of dyslexia I have been
involved with the Dyslexia Institute, run by Mrs Wendy
Fisher, for even longer. The Dyslexia Institute has concentrated on diagnosing dyslexia through psychological tests
and starting special teaching centres throughout the
country. With the help of the Institute and Grenville
College, and Dr Ifor Capel, we analysed hair samples from
seventy-seven British dyslexic children. The dyslexic
children had an average of twenty-five times more cadmium
in their hair than control children and higher copper and
aluminium levels. About 81 per cent of the dyslexics had
detectable cadmium compared with 25 per cent of the

159

controls. Both controls and dyslexics had low zinc and high lead levels.[14]

Over the past ten years fifty-one studies have been published showing that children with behavioural or learning difficulties have more toxic metals in their hair, especially cadmium and lead, and abnormalities of the essential nutritional elements.[15] Unfortunately, however, hair testing has fallen under a cloud because it can give such variable results for essential nutritional elements especially zinc. Zinc is one of the most important elements for the developing brain and efficient brain functioning but zinc deficiency in our society is almost universal. When the body's zinc is really low, hair growth tends to slow and the levels of zinc and toxic metals tend to rise in hair. Severe zinc deficiency can however exist with a hair test showing low, normal or high zinc readings.

Dr Lodge Rees and Mrs Barnes allowed for this by advising all patients or would-be parents to take extra zinc and vitamin C, which they recommend for reducing the body's toxic metal overload by encouraging the excretion of toxic metals.

My own experience of this confusing anomaly was a very abnormal hair test from an eleven-year-old dyslexic boy called Malcolm. He had reading, writing and spelling difficulties and poor concentration. He was unable to keep still for any length of time. The hair test showed high zinc, high copper and some toxic metals. He reacted to supplements, however, with diarrhoea, perhaps because they contained yeast, and refused to continue to take them. A year later he became depressed, listless and anorexic. He was no longer hyperactive. By then I had heard that Dr John Howard was carrying out more detailed mineral analysis at the London Clinic. Besides hair, he was also testing blood and sweat as he had discovered that the sweat analysis gave a much more accurate reading of body zinc status than either the hair or the blood readings. While the hair zinc is confused by the speed of hair growth, the blood zinc is controlled by regulating mechanisms.

Dr Stephen Davies, one of the clinical ecology doctors, collaborated with Dr Howard and they found that zinc supplementation brought the sweat zinc back to normal. This could take up to three months in cases of severe deficiency. [16]

Once more my dyslexic patient had high hair zinc but his sweat zinc was well below the normal range and so was his magnesium and chromium. This time supplements and a low allergy diet produced such a dramatic improvement that one of his teachers accompanied Malcolm and his mother making their follow-up visit to tell me how delighted she was with his schoolwork and behaviour. Malcolm had won the class prize for the greatest improvement — and also for spelling!

Zinc in Pregnancy

The average British diet is said to contain 10mg of elemental zinc while the average daily requirement is officially estimated at a conservative 15mg a day. Pregnant women require 20mg but lactating mothers need 25mg a day. A breast-fed baby reaches adult zinc status by three months old but a bottle-fed baby takes six months. Baby boys are especially liable to zinc deficiency which, together with toxic metals, is a major cause of susceptibility to food allergies leading to infantile colic and eczema. The best sources of zinc are oysters and red meat. Some young women on the pill become intolerant to meat however, and thus run the risk of developing zinc deficiency.

The recent high fibre diet craze can upset the absorption of zinc so that it is best to take zinc tablets or drops last thing at night if cereals are taken in the morning. For many years now there has also been a practice of prescribing iron, in far too large doses, for pregnant women, but iron antagonises zinc and prevents absorption. If iron is needed, small amounts should be taken early in the day. The safest sources are the natural ones as direct iron supplementation may give rise to unwanted side-effects.

Foresight has worked out a programme of mineral and vitamin supplementation based on hair analysis monitoring for parents-to-be, pregnant and lactating mothers and children. Two Foresight mineral and vitamin tablets a day are equivalent in essential nutrients to two good meals a day.

Belinda Barnes has collaborated with Irene Colquhoun of the Hyperactive Children's Support Group to publish *The Hyperactive Child — What the Family Can Do*. This book describes the rationale behind a simple self-help programme.[17]

The latest Foresight research is being carried out by Professor Derek Bryce-Smith at Reading. He is comparing the trace minerals in samples from areas of high neonatal mortality (Merseyside, Barnsley and South Wales) with samples from low risk areas (Oxford, and East Crete in Greece). This work is a follow-on to his previously published results that children who are born dead for no apparent reason had ten times more lead and cadmium in their bones than children who died for known reasons. These unexpected stillbirths also had low levels of zinc and calcium.[18] The Reading team are now analysing thirty-six elements in nine different tissue samples taken from 500 normal and abnormal births. The early results show that the placenta provides no significant barrier to the toxic metals from the mother reaching the fetus.

Small, premature low birth weight babies, who are also much more likely than full-sized term babies to have abnormalities not only have significantly more toxic metals — lead, cadmium, aluminium or mercury — but also have significantly less zinc. Small babies are also especially likely to have copper in toxic amounts. Small amounts of copper are needed for normal full-term growth but high levels of copper act like the toxic metals and displace zinc.

Several researchers, notably Professor Lucille Hurley, University of California,[19] have shown that zinc deficiency in pregnant rats can cause stillbirths and birth defects.

Professor Donald Oberleas[20] and others discovered that if baby rats are short of zinc they are unable to find their way out of a maze, but that they quickly learn the correct path when they are fed extra zinc. If, however, their mother was kept short of zinc during her pregnancy, giving the babies extra is no help. They are never able to learn which path leads to the food.

This is an immensely valuable piece of research because it means we may not always be able to put the clock back. The mother's health before and during early pregnancy is of the utmost importance. Diet and supplementation may help children in later life but may not be able to restore them to their full intellectual capacity which was their hereditary birth right. This not only applies to learning difficulties but also to behaviour problems and to the development of a normal immune system.[21] Lack of adequate dietary zinc during pregnancy and lactation, the two critical periods, may lead to a marked immuno-deficiency which can be remarkably persistent, even with long-term nutritional rehabilitation. In animal studies, if the parents are malnourished the health of the children can be adversely affected for several generations.

Declining Intelligence

At a recent conference on mineral analysis I met Dr Bernard Rimland, a psychologist working for the American Navy. Dr Rimland has investigated the apparent decline in the quality of new recruits. One report had estimated that in 1980 the Navy was short of 20,000 personnel for its middle grade skilled jobs. After complaints from field commanders and training personnel, Dr Rimland reviewed the evidence.[22]

Throughout the United States college-bound high school leavers are assessed by the Scholastic Aptitude Test (SAT). Between 1953 and 1963 these average scores stayed the same with males showing superior mathematical ability but both sexes having similar verbal scores. For the next seventeen years all the scores plunged downwards. By 1980 the maths score declined 36 points to 466 and the verbal score dropped 54 points to 424. The scores are lower now than ever before in their fifty-one-year history. The number of very high scoring students has declined even more drastically and Dr Rimland says top universities now compete for top scorers with the same enthusiasm that they used to reserve for football players.

There is also a striking, almost mirror-image correlation between the decline in SAT scores and the increase in violent crime. Dr Rimland thinks this correlation is so strong that it suggests one or more common causes. He also shows that as expenditure in education increased so educational achievement continued to decline unabated.

There are many possible reasons for this decline, pollution, nuclear fall-out, smoking, alcoholism, drugs and chemicals, but the use of the birth control pill and other hormones are especially mentioned as there is evidence that a single exposure to such substances can trigger a permanent change in the child's brain and endocrine system. Not only is a child at grave risk if the mother inadvertently or deliberately takes hormones in early pregnancy, but pill use induces mineral imbalance — especially low zinc and high copper. Women who have just stopped the pill, even if they are having good diets, are likely to be zinc deficient.

The zinc requirements are high in pregnancy but, unfortunately, taking extra zinc is not yet generally advised. Even if a woman waits six months or longer before becoming pregnant, it is still unlikely that she will have an adequate zinc intake unless she takes extra.

Zinc supplementation is remarkably safe but prolonged use of very high doses (60mg elemental zinc daily), which are used in the treatment of depression or schizophrenia, can cause an iron or copper deficiency anaemia which quickly responds to taking extra iron or copper. Usually, however, we tend to have plenty of copper as our water supply collects copper as it travels through copper pipes. Women who have used the pill, or a copper IUD or smoked, are very likely to have copper levels in the high toxic range. The highest copper levels Foresight have found in hair have been in women using IUDs.

Congenital Abnormalities

With up to 50 per cent of pregnant women smoking, and increasing alcoholism among young women, it is difficult to find out what is the statistical risk of having an abnormal baby if you have ever used the pill. It is also now known that if the father is zinc deficient and smokes or drinks he is more likely to produce abnormal sperm. It has been known since 1967[23] that the pill increases the risk of chromosome abnormalities and a 1979 paper reported significantly higher rates of sister-chromatid exchanges among women taking 'low-dose' pills compared with normal and pregnant women.[24] As women get older they have an increased risk of chromosome abnormalities. Professor Lejeune in Paris questioned mothers of 730 children with Down's Syndrome and found those over thirty were significantly more likely to have used the pill for longer than one year and/or to have become pregnant within six months of stopping it.[25]

The Oxford/FPA study reported the results of 5,700 pregnancies and found 'a surprisingly low incidence' of congenital abnormalities among live infants born to women having their first baby who had never taken the pill. The figures were 0.4 per cent compared with 3.8 per cent in 1976 and 0.9 per cent compared with 4.3 per cent in 1979.[26]

The 1974 RCGP report listed a higher risk of abortion among women stopping the pill. The 193 women who had stopped the pill to get pregnant had an abortion rate of 13.37 per cent which was similar to the rate in controls but the 349 women discontinuing for other reasons, presumably mostly side-effects, had an abortion rate of 30.61 per cent compared with 12.28 per cent in controls. The authors speculated that these women were more likely to have induced abortions.

But Dr Isobel Gal had already found out that the incidence of malformations was usually three times higher in induced abortions and ten times higher in spontaneous abortions than in total births.[27] She says that female hormones are powerful teratogens (substances likely to cause congenital abnormalities) in animals in all phases of reproduction and although oestrogen is thought to be more harmful than progesterone preparations, changes in balance may be important. Dr Gal had discovered, in 1967, that women who had used hormone pregnancy tests had a much higher risk of having a baby with spina bifida or other central nervous system malformation.[28] By an almost single-handed campaign she succeeded in having hormone pregnancy tests banned in the UK and in most developed countries. Registration for spina bifida began in 1968 and the incidence has fallen from a peak in 1972. Sometimes doses equivalent to nine months of oral contraceptive use were given in early pregnancy at a time when the fetus is at its most vulnerable. Dr Gal is very concerned about the morning-after contraceptive pill — which is a bigger than usual dose of hormones. The current advice is that if a pregnancy continues after hormones have been used unsuccessfully to induce an abortion, the pregnancy should be terminated surgically.

There is no argument now that exposure to exogenous hormones in pregnancy increases a woman's chances of an abnormal baby. The American husband and wife team, Nora and Nora, checked back the histories of babies born with multiple abnormalities including limb-reduction defects, like the Thalidomide children, and discovered that out of thirty cases, half had been exposed to oestrogen/progesterone preparations. Of the others, three had been exposed to alcohol, two X-rays, one anaesthetics and the rest various drugs or severe infections.[29] Hormone exposure in early pregnancy increases the risk of limb defects by twenty-three times.[30] Professor Janerich and others also reported an increase in limb-reduction defects but W. F. Robertson described in 1962[31] how riboflavin deficiency, vitamin B2, may be one of the causes of the Thalidomide tragedies. My colleague, Professor Capel, discovered more recently that young women taking low dose pills have abnormally high levels of glutathione peroxidase after seven months of low dose pills, and as the levels of the enzyme go up, the red blood cell levels of riboflavin go down. This important fault in metabolism can remain after stopping the pill and is not corrected, experimentally, by taking vitamin B2.[32]

Many authors have reported an increased risk of abnormalities including increased cardio-vascular abnormalities and Rothman found an increase in spontaneous abortion, stillbirth and twinning among previous pill users.

The picture is confused by the increase in smoking by young women since the last war. In 1979 half of the pregnant mothers in Cardiff were smoking. When I reviewed the effects of smoking and the pill for a Foresight meeting in 1980, I discovered that they were similar. Both cause upsets in liver function and minerals and vitamins. Smokers have higher plasma proteins with raised ceruloplasmin concentrations and high copper. As both copper and cadmium, from cigarettes, antagonise zinc, smokers and pill takers are usually zinc deficient and therefore more susceptible to the toxic effects of lead pollution.[12] Smokers have lower vitamin A, and up to 30 to 40 per cent lower vitamin C levels than non-smokers. Vitamin B12 may be lowered as it is necessary for cyanide metabolism.

Smoking damages the placenta, and is the major cause of small babies due to lack of zinc and high toxic metals. Because smokers are more likely to abort a normal fetus than are either non-smokers or oral contraceptive users, it was thought at first that smoking was not teratogenic. However, recent studies found smokers were more likely to have babies with all types of congenital abnormalities, especially cleft palate, hare lip, facial malformations, squint and heart and brain abnormalities.

If a woman has been exposed to toxic substances her

pregnancies may be affected in a number of ways.

1. She may be infertile. Alcoholic women tend not to conceive.
2. She may abort early and the fetus may be normal or abnormal.
3. She may give birth to an obviously abnormal child.
4. She may have an apparently normal looking child who later develops behaviour problems, learning difficulties, or is very allergic with a reduced ability to cope with stress.
5. She may have a normal child.

Some fetuses seem to be immune from toxic effects. Even a mother who is severely alcoholic may produce a normal looking baby. A case has been described when one twin showed the characteristics of the full-blown fetal alcohol syndrome at birth while the other twin looked normal.

Again, as the pill causes mineral and vitamin imbalance and liver function changes, the effects of any alcohol a woman takes are likely to be increased.

Long Term Effects in Women

Perhaps the most chilling account of long-term effects of hormone exposure on women's ovaries and future children has been described by Professor Jean Jofen, a New York psychologist.[33] She discovered that some Jewish children of very intelligent parents had unexpectedly severe learning defects with IQs between 80 and 100. She discovered a common factor. All of their mothers had been held captive during the war in the same concentration camp — Auschwitz. She did not find the same problem when mothers had been in other concentration camps, suggesting that starvation alone was not the cause. Women who had gone to Auschwitz had stopped menstruating within ten days of their arrival. Hunger and stress take longer than that to affect the human system which has reserves of fat especially to cater for such emergencies. None of the mothers remembered any medical treatment or injections but some thought the soup had been 'treated'. Eventually Professor Jofen unearthed a secret document among the Nuremberg trial records. Greenhouses had been built in Auschwitz to grow a rare South American plant from which female hormones could be made. These were 'to lead to sterilisation of persons without their knowledge'.

The really chilling part of the story is that it was the women who were permanently affected. The men of Auschwitz later had children with normal IQs. And yet we are witnessing in the 1980s a social scene where smoking, drinking, pill taking and even drug addiction are becoming commonplace among younger and younger girls. Professor Jofen had found that *the lower the child's IQ was, the younger the mother had been when she was first introduced to hormones*. Not all facets of intelligence were affected equally which is a typical finding among dyslexic children.

Although a Japanese chemical company developed a profitable new microbial method for making the pill from cholesterol, the Japanese Welfare Ministry was not prepared to lift the ban on the use of this type of contraceptive because of its ability to cause cancer and congenital abnormalities. Japan is famous among the world's 'rich' countries for having a low animal fat diet and an exceptionally low incidence of breast cancer. They are also beginning to lead the world in original scientific research.

Professor Jofen thought the best place to check on the pill's effect on children would be Puerto Rico where the pill was first used on a large scale. But the official, expensive and perfectly designed control trial carried out on 9,757 women between 1961 and 1976 came up with nothing — even the women taking the original high dose oestrogen pills had no statistical increase in thrombosis, metabolic upsets or cancer. Perhaps the fact that by 1976 only twenty-six active pill users were followed up might have something to do with these results. [34]

169

Precocious Sexual Development

Not everyone, however, is happy about Puerto Rico's children. During 1978 and 1981 there was a striking increase in the incidence of precocious sexual development in children from as young as age six months to eight years.[35] Dr Carmen Rodrigues, a paediatrician, came to London to lecture at the Royal Society of Medicine in 1984. She showed picture after picture of children with breast and sexual development — of girls who had started to menstruate at the same time that they had first started school and of boys who were also developing too soon. She suspected the oestrogenic substances, stilboestrol and zeranol, which are freely available in Puerto Rico and are used to improve the growth weight of chickens. Dr Schoental wrote to the *Lancet* that oestrogens in the pill could have added to the natural oestrogens like zeralenone in food and influenced the children perinatally so that they were more likely to be sensitive to hormones in food. In the same year, at a Clinical Ecology conference in Torquay, it was reported that 6 per cent of American children tested reacted positively to skin titrations for progesterone. How have these children become allergic to their natural hormones?

Birth Marks

A large study of 16,000 women in Jerusalem in 1978[36] had found that there were significantly more children with skin vascular abnormalities (birthmarks) if their mothers had got pregnant immediately after stopping the pill compared with those who had become pregnant after waiting for one or more months. Women who were over thirty-five or who were underweight or who had become pregnant immediately had an increased risk of a miscarriage or an abnormal baby. Since that study it has been generally recommended that women should wait at least three months before becoming pregnant.

170

Spina Bifida

Dr Isobel Gal was working for the Medical Research Council when she discovered that women taking the pill had high plasma levels of vitamin A. During the first three months after stopping the pill, the vitamin A levels did gradually fall but they did not all return to normal levels.[37] Dr Gal found mothers of spina bifida children were more likely to have very high vitamin A levels. Abnormal babies also had high liver vitamin A concentrations.

The rise in blood vitamin A may be because the pill raises plasma proteins and vitamin A is transported attached to gamma-globulin. Animal studies have shown that vitamin A accumulates in the liver when there is zinc deficiency. Because of regulatory mechanisms, blood vitamin A levels only alter when there is an extreme excess or deficiency of vitamin A. Either too high or too low levels can cause fetal abnormalities. Vitamin E is also needed for adequate vitamin A uptake as it prevents the oxidation of fats. But the pill may interfere with fat metabolism and leads to a shortage of gamma linolenic acid (GLA).

Essential Fats

The brain and the central nervous system are formed from essential fatty acids. Especially important is linoleic acid which is present in vegetable oils such as sunflower, corn and olive oils. To be active, linoleic acid needs to be converted to gamma linolenic acid. Women with premenstrual tension or breast lumps and hyperactive or dyslexic children all seem especially susceptible to GLA deficiency and benefit from evening primrose oil supplements. This is the only natural oil apart from human milk which contains the vital GLA. Men with heart disease are also GLA deficient, probably mostly due to smoking or drinking.

Normally linoleic acid, in the diet, is converted to GLA with the help of zinc, the B vitamins and vitamin C. I have already explained, that as part of the upset in antioxidant glutathione metabolism, riboflavin falls with pill use, but taking hormones also lowers levels of vitamin C and other B complex vitamins including folic acid and vitamin B12; while changes in cortisol and amine metabolism can cause vitamin B6 deficiency.

Through animal studies it has been well-known for many years that excesses or deficiencies of minerals and vitamins can cause most kinds of fetal abnormalities. In 1980 Professor R. W. Smithells and his team[38] described a reduction in neural tube defect incidence of from 5 per cent to 0.6 per cent when mothers who had previously had babies with this abnormality were given a multivitamin preparation and iron (but no extra zinc) for at least one month before conception. The very act of leaving a gap between stopping the pill and conceiving would also help.

Sick Children

We are witnessing a sharp increase in childhood problems — babies and children with severe allergies to cow's milk or wheat, and, besides the epidemic of hyperactivity, more and more of our children are growing up unable to learn to read, write or count.

Cot deaths (sudden unexplained deaths during sleep) more than doubled during the seventies and now kill one in 500 infants up to two years old.[39] While infants are now less likely to die from infections, the unexplained deaths have increased from one in ten to one in three. Cot deaths happen in all social class families, suggesting a new cause more important than nutrition, housing, hygiene or even smoking and it seems not unreasonable to suggest that maternal hormone exposure may play a part.

The increased risks to our children do not end in infancy. The estimated suicide rate for both boys and girls has increased by 50 per cent over the past ten years.[40] Not only are children now more likely to be victims of marital

172

disharmony and maternal psychiatric disturbances, but accidental or deliberate exposure to hormones during pregnancy or at birth can cause persistent changes in brain control and immunity. Hormones have been given freely and extravagantly to younger and younger women, but at what cost?

Sexually Transmitted Diseases

Infections of the genital organs, historically known as venereal diseases, are spread by sexual contact with an infected person. Now known as Sexually Transmitted Diseases (STD), new cases have increased by nearly 600 per cent since the pill and the greatest increases have been in women and teenagers.

It was very clear from the large pill studies that pill users had more infections of all types including sexually transmitted diseases. Even if steroid hormones did not compromise a woman's immune system, the trend has been to give the pill to younger and younger girls before they are physically, emotionally or mentally ready for a mature permanent relationship so that the number of partners men and women chalk up has gone on increasing. This, of course, is the best way to spread VD. The new attendances at STD clinics in Britain[41] rose from less than 100,000 per year in the late 1950s to an all time high of 562,841 in 1982. There have been large increases in candidiasis (56,126), herpes (14,836), genital warts (37,334), lice (10,900) and non-specific genital infections (142,066). After also dramatically increasing there have been recent falls in new cases of syphilis and gonorrhoea. Both of these can usually be treated with penicillin, but there have been increases in resistant strains. The true incidence of STDs is much higher as under reporting is widespread.

Yeast or Candida

It is virtually impossible for a husband and wife to infect each other with most VDs such as syphilis or gonorrhoea if they have never had sex with anyone else. An exception is *candidiasis*, which is also known as thrush or monilia. Thrush is caused by the yeast candida albicans, a normal inhabitant of our digestive tract but it can overgrow and cause irritating white plaques in the vagina when a woman's resistance is lowered by taking the pill, antibiotics, repeated pregnancies, or eating too much sugar, yeast or carbohydrate. Candidiasis is at least doubled among pill users and it can cause allergies to foods and chemicals and even severe mental illness. Treatment of systemic candidiasis has been described as 'a medical breakthrough'. Yeast allergy is extremely common and underdiagnosed.[42]

Pelvic Inflamatory Disease (PID)

Non specific genital infections, which include chlamydia trachomatis, are the commonest STDs diagnosed at special clinics. Chlamydia, like gonorrhoea, commonly produces no signs or symptoms in women but has been discovered in 31 per cent of women attending STD clinics.

Both chlamydia and gonorrhoea are very serious infections as they are major causes of *pelvic inflamatory disease* (PID) which is developed by 10 per cent of STD patients.[43] The infections can spread through the uterus, along the tubes and into the pelvic cavity. The long term consequences can be chronic abdominal pain, menstrual disturbances, dyspareunia (painful intercourse), infertility, tubal pregnancy and sterility. The proportion of patients with infected tubes who develop tubal blockage rises from 12.8 per cent with the first attack to 75 per cent with three or more. The number of severe cases admitted to hospital has doubled in the past 20 years. In the United States the direct costs of such admissions is estimated at $400 million a year.

In some African countries up to 45 per cent of all gynaecological admissions are due to PID. A woman with a mixed infection of gonorrhoea and chlamydia has a 50 per cent chance of a relapse, a 25 per cent chance of dyspareunia , a one in three chance of becoming sterile and a 10 per cent chance of an ectopic pregnancy. The sharpest increase in PID was between 1976 and 1980 when the number of younger women using the pill and the IUD increased.

The three main pill studies, using mostly older married women showed immediate increase in many infections including STDs between 1968 and 1972.

The 1974 RCGP report listed statistically significant increases among pill users including colds, respiratory infections, influenza, rhinitis, sinusitus and pleurisy. Urinary infections, cervicitis, cervical erosions, vaginitis, monilia, trichomoniasis, leukorrhoea (white discharge) and pruritis (itch) of the genital organs were also increased. While there were 1,115 cases of vaginal thrush among pill users (rate 31.46) and only 661 cases among the controls (rate 15.89), there were 15 cases (rate 0.42) of PID among pill takers but 36 (rate 0.89) among controls. There was then massive and repeated publicity that the pill reduced the risk of PID by half — not mentioning, of course, that women who had stopped the pill had higher rates than those who had never taken the pill (rate 1.02).

Women joining the Walnut Creek study who had ever used the pill had significantly more thrush, trichomonas, discharge or itching, cervicitis, PID (infection of the tubes), infection of the uterus and gonorrhoea. During the period of observation pill users had more urinary tract infections. Past users had significant increases in almost all the conditions of the genital tract studied including pelvic peritoneal adhesions which can lead to sterility.

Pill users joining the Oxford/FPA study had more vaginitis and cervicitis than either diaphragm or IUD users. During the survey IUD users had three times more PID and infected tubes than either the pill or diaphragm users, but the total numbers were small.

Since then many case control studies have claimed that current pill use reduces PID but there is a shortage of normal controls. IUD use increases PID and so does having multiple partners. Recently, a quarter of teenagers attending an STD clinic were not using a reliable contraceptive although they had been sexually active for as long or longer with a larger number of partners than the contraceptive users. They were several times more likely to have caught gonorrhoea.

Studies comparing such irresponsible teenagers with pill users would give an erroneous impression that pill use protected against PID as Oliver Gillie, medical correspondent of the *Sunday Times* pointed out to me. There seems to be no doubt that pill use increases the infections that lead to PID although a woman may not be diagnosed until she has already stopped taking the pill.

Unfortunately PID is difficult to diagnose and may be confused with appendicitis, endometriosis (where endometrial tissue grows around in the pelvis) and ectopic pregnancy.

As many STDs are asymptomatic in women, gonorrhoea or chlamydia are commonly only diagnosed when female contacts of men suffering from sexual diseases are routinely investigated and yet their long term consequences are far greater for women.

Ectopic Pregnancies

An egg sometimes implants outside the uterus, in the tube or in the pelvis. These ectopic pregnancies have increased in the U.S. from 6.5 to 21.7 per 1000 conceptions in the past ten years. This increase matches the increase in STD and especially infection with chlamydia trachomatis, which has been found in 69 per cent of cases. Known as the 'quiet epidemic', chlamydia infections damage the tubes progressively and silently increasing the chance of an ectopic pregnancy which, in turn, often leads to the loss of a fallopian tube. The increase in ectopic pregnancies is also linked with increase in maternal age, IUD use and induced abortions. An acute attack of PID increases the risk of an ectopic pregnancy six times.

Genital Wart Virus Infection

Obvious genital warts have doubled in frequency in the past eight years. Until recently they were regarded as merely a nuisance but now they are thought to be responsible for a sinister and alarming epidemic — a rapidly progressive form of cervical cancer in young women.[44] A third of women examined with a colposcope have evidence of a human papilloma virus (HPV) lesion on their cervix and nearly all cervical premalignant lesions are infected with the virus. There is evidence that the pill, smoking and herpes act together with the HPV wart virus to increase the development of early invisible cervical cancers. Both oestrogen and progesterone increase small DNA tumour virus polyomas in mouse tissue culture. Vulvar warts tend to increase in pregnancy but the horrific increase in early cervical cancer in young women began when the pill was introduced.

Damage to Babies

Antibiotics have had a spectacular impact on the long term effects of syphilis and congentital syphilis has become very rare, but the new generation of STDs including the virus infections are now affecting thousands of babies every year.[45]

Herpes

Herpes is the most common cause of genital ulceration in the UK. The infections cause recurrent painful ulcers, interfere with the sufferer's sex life and are highly infectious, readily transferring from person to person. If a mother has an active

177

attack during delivery the baby is likely to be infected. In 1978 it was estimated that 740 babies died of herpes and 180 suffered permanent neurological damage. There may be damage to the baby's eyes, skin or liver. Treatment is unsatisfactory and infection with herpes may be a life-long sentence.[43] Several studies have linked antenatal viral infection with subsequent malignant disease.

Cytomegalovirus

If the first infection with this virus happens during pregnancy, the baby can have brain damage, blindness, deafness, microcephaly (small head), mental retardation, cerebral palsy or even die. The virus is mainly sexually transmitted but is also found in saliva. Prenatal infections affect thousands of babies and one to two per cent will have a severe disease. In the UK it is estimated that about 2,800 babies are infected annually, and at lease 500 have severe brain damage.

Another common sexually transmitted virus is the hepatitis B virus which is an important cause of liver damage resulting in an increase in food and chemical allergies in a mother. If a woman has allergic reactions to common foods, these can affect her baby and cause infantile colic when she is breast feeding.

Chlamydia

This important and often silent bacterial infection can cause conjunctivitis in the new-born baby's eyes. In San Francisco over five per cent of new born babies are infected during delivery. Erythromycin or tetracycline eye ointments cure the eye disease but they do not prevent chlamidial pneumonia, which accounts for 30 per cent of all cases of pneumonia in infants under six months of age.

Multiple Infections

In a review of 115 pregnant inner-city adolescents age 13 to 17 in Baltimore, the incidence of multiple STDs was very high.[46] Thirty-eight per cent had candida and 37 per cent chlamydia trachomatis. These infections alone did not effect the pregnancy outcome. Trichomonas vaginalis infected 34 per cent, mycoplasma hominis 70 per cent and ureaplasma urealyticum from 90 per cent. Some also had gonorrhoea. Cervical infection with trichomonas was associated with lower gestational age and weight at birth. Mothers infected with both chlamydia trachomatis and trichomonas had the smallest babies. Some mothers, delivered by caesarian section had inflamation of the lining of the womb after delivery. Among 90 infants 11 had conjunctivitis, 27 upper respiratory infections and four had pneumonia in the first four months of life. There was one stillbirth.

The Acquired Immune Deficiency Syndrome AIDS

AIDS, unknown when the first cases were described in 1981, is causing a panic in California. In four years over 16,000 Americans have developed AIDS and half of them have died. In the U.K. the total number of cases had reached 206 with 114 deaths up to August 1985. It is estimated that half a million people in the U.S. and 10,000 in the U.K. are infected with the HTLV III virus which causes AIDS. The interval between infection and clinical AIDS is known to vary from a few months to as long as five years. As many as 10 per cent of those infected may develop the serious form of the disease. It has been described as the 'new plague' — the 'new black death' and 'the blight of our future'.

A massive publicity campaign is being launched to educate homosexuals and drug abusers about unsafe practices. The virus has been isolated from blood, semen and saliva. Almost a quarter of high risk homosexuals tested in 1985 had antibodies to the virus which show up in the blood two weeks to four months after infection.[47]

Infertility

There have already been reports of women being infected by the AIDS virus after receiving AID — artificial insemination from donors. Some of my Foresight couples have expressed concern about this. In 24 per cent of couples suffering from infertility, the cause is found to be sperm defects. But sperm counts can be used as a test of zinc levels. Low sperm counts often reflect low zinc levels in sweat and zinc supplementation can give excellent results for infertile couples so that they no longer need to resort to AID.

In-vitro fertilisation is now being used for women who have blocked fallopian tubes.

Mrs A became infertile after using a copper IUD for two years. Investigations over several years showed her tubes had become irreparably damaged by infections (PID). She waited a year to reach the top of the in-vitro fertilisation waiting list which then cost her over £2,000. She had noticed white spots on her finger nails and having read that this was a sign of zinc deficiency she started to take zinc sulphate. When she went to the hospital she was told to stop taking the zinc. Five ova were obtained after her ovaries had been artificially stimulated by brain hormones but none of the eggs managed to implant. When I tested her minerals a few weeks later her sweat zinc was consistent with a marked deficiency. Zinc deficiency may be one reason why the in-vitro fertilisation programme is not always successful.

Another important point is age; fertility falls off with age and many couples now use contraception for 10 or 20 years before starting their families when they are in their late 30s or early 40s.

It is estimated that one in six couples have infertility problems at some time — that is — failing to conceive within two and a half years. It is not surprising as severe zinc deficiency is so common — due to nutritionally inadequate

180

diets with vegetarians and vegans at special risk. The pill or IUD, smoking and alcohol or food allergies or candida or toxic metal contamination, all increase the likelihood of zinc deficiency. Of infertile couples investigated by the NHS 21 per cent have ovulation failure, 14 per cent have tubal damage which has a poor treatment success rate unless IVF is used, 24 per cent have sperm defects and 28 per cent are unexplained by traditional means.[48]

It is Forsight's experience that many unexplained cases of sperm defects and ovulation failure cases are due to upsets in minerals. Change of habits, diet and adding nutritional supplements produces such quick results that we have to warn infertile couples to use some method of contraception until their mineral analysis has become stabilised back into the normal range. Dr John Howard has found that if a woman starts pregnancy with a normal sweat zinc she can be maintained with a minimal supplementation and does not experience a fall in her zinc status. The aim of Foresight is to correct serious deficiencies or excesses before conception takes place. Repeated miscarriages also have similar causes with low magnesium as well as low zinc usually found. A sad, if not tragic conflict has developed in the medical journals about zinc status in pregnancy. The conflict has arisen because blood zinc tends to be held in the normal range by control mechanisms while hair zinc may be low, normal or high in zinc deficient states.[49] The sweat test, first used in 1949, is excellent and we have found that nearly all the 45 dyslexic children we tested had below normal levels of zinc in their sweat. Only one little boy had a low blood zinc and his sweat zinc was the lowest of all the children tested. He was hyperactive and violent to his classmates, his mother was also seriously zinc deficient and had recently had a stillbirth.

In September 1985 an editorial in the *British Journal of Obstetrics and Gynaecology* said that 'nature has perfected the most bizarre diagnostic trap: an illusion in which normal masquerades as abnormal'.

The editor contended, mostly on the evidence from one

Medical Research Council study,[50] that low blood zinc is normal in pregnancy and that there is no evidence for giving zinc supplements to pregnant women. The MRC group measured plasma, hair and urine zinc levels in Hindu and European pregnant women, all had low zinc intakes (3.1 to 16.9 mg per day), well below the recommended intake for pregnancy. The Hindu vegetarians had the lowest intakes. 34 per cent of the Hindu babies were light-for-dates but only six per cent of the European babies, even though a third of their mothers continued to smoke.

The average zinc blood levels were below the Biolab normal range (11.5 to 20 micromols/litre) throughout the pregnancies. Dr John Howard of Biolab has found that when zinc intake is adequate during pregnancy the blood levels do not fall below normal, although the copper levels still increase above this normal range (12.5 to 25 micromols/litre) due to the high oestrogen production in pregnancy. The conclusions of the MRC paper was that there was no evidence that the lower average zinc status of the Hindus, who had significant lower blood zinc and higher copper than the European mothers, had 'acted as a nutritional constraint' or was the cause of their slower rate of intra uterine growth.

What then was the cause of the 'famine' pattern of poor growth and so many small babies?

The reality is that the pill causes zinc deficiency. When women on very low zinc diets take oral contraceptives they enter a vicious circle of declining health. The pill may alter the actions of the zinc and dependent enzymes in the gut lining and absorption of zinc and other minerals can be impaired — leading to further zinc deficiency and yeast or candida overgrowth releasing fungal toxins causing more allergies and reactions to carbohydrates and sugar.[42] Unless steps are taken to correct these abnormalities before pregnancy many women become pregnant in a state of biochemical upset. However if the mineral balance is stabilised before pregnancy, women can be maintained during pregnancy with small doses of supplements such as two Foresight minerals and vitamins each day.

It is tragic that, so far, the medical establishment is continuing to ignore or deny the links between oral contraceptive use and the increasing problems in fertility, pregnancy and the number of congenital abnormalities. A very high number of early pregnancies end in miscarriage and at least one in seven pregnancies have less than an ideal outcome — clearly much too high a figure for a well fed, civilised and scientific society.

It is now estimated that nearly a half of London's school children have problems with basic learning skills, reading, writing and arithmetic at age 15. Many animal studies clearly show that zinc is essential for brain development and function[51] and our dyslexia study has confirmed the importance of THINK ZINC.

Professor Bryce Smith, whose studies on placentae have shown the importance of zinc for intra uterine growth, has devised a simple cheap test for zinc deficiency.[52a,b]

Zinc Taste Test

Two teaspoonfuls of a 0.1 per cent solution of zinc sulphate hepta hydrate are tasted.

The responses can be graded:
1. No taste after 5 to 10 seconds = severe zinc deficiency.
2. Slightly dry taste after 5 to 10 seconds = moderate zinc deficiency
3. Immediate taste = mild zinc deficiency
4. Unpleasant taste producing a strong grimace = adequate zinc status.

The sweat test needs expensive equipment, meticulous analysis and an hour's visit to the laboratory but the diagnosis and treatment of mineral abnormalities could result in untold benefits to future generations.

But we are at the second generation of pill takers. Anorexia has become a cult disease. The sufferers are usually

183

teenage girls with severe zinc deficiency and their appetite returns when they are given zinc sulphate.

We had already found that these girls had abnormal fast liver clearance and abnormal copper to zinc ratios at Charing Cross Hospital in 1978. A new type of ovarian disease, with multiple cysts, has been described,[53] especially common in anorexics during weight gain. The ovaries become normal when the weight returns to normal. There are higher risks to babies among women conceiving at a low weight. Ultrasonographic examination[54] showed all 19 healthy young women taking a low dose contraceptive pill had multiple ovarian follicules on their seventh pill free day, making conception quite likely if they forgot to take a pill. This confirms our early work showing the higher pregnancy risk of low dose pills.

In contrast an Israeli study[55] of 64 teenages (average age 18.3) found 34.3 per cent were not ovulating when they were requesting oral contraception. Has regular ovulation always been this late or is it a second generation effect? Either way this study emphasises it may be unnecessary to give many teenagers an ovulation blocking drug when they are not ovulating but, even more importantly, normal ovarian stimulation is being interfered with at a time of great natural change and sensitivity. The normal Biolab range of sweat copper for girls increases from the childhood and male range of 400—900 to 420—1410 after the onset of menstruation. Interfering with such basic mechanisms is lunacy.

Summary

* Hormones during pregnancy can cause:
  sexual abnormalities — males can be feminised and females can be masculinised
  vaginal cancer in girls and testicular cancer in young men

* 1 in 250 boys have some abnormality in their external genitals and 1 in 10 have undescended testes at birth.

Each year more boys than girls are being born with obvious congenital abnormalities

* Hormones before pregnancy can cause upsets to vitamins and minerals in the mother increasing the risk of congenital abnormalities, behaviour problems and learning difficulties

* Today's babies are more likely to die unexpectedly in their cots

* Today's teenagers are more likely to be promiscuous, have more STDs and girls are more likely to have abortions

* There is an increase in teenage pregnancies outside marriage

* Today's mothers are more likely to be in their 30s and be zinc deficient

* Sweat test or zinc taste test can diagnose zinc deficiency and treatment can alleviate many of the pill-induced problems

9 *The Future Beckons*

This is a story full of optimism and pessimism. The optimism springs from the fact that we can accurately identify a source of illness in the world; the pessimism by our stubborn reluctance to deal with it. Women themselves cannot forever duck out of this issue. They cannot go on opting for the simplicity of a chemical contraceptive until it damages their health and then blame everyone but themselves. To embark voluntarily on a continuing course of therapy without first understanding what bodily mechanisms are likely to be involved is a kind of irresponsibility not worthy of the modern woman. The only group of women I spare from this criticism is the very young, who are racing into sexual adventures earlier than the last generation, and being initiated into contraceptive 'drugtaking' before they are of an age when they can give truly considered consent. Doctors should resist the pressure to prescribe the pill for them. The medical profession needs to unite against steroids in the same way it is belatedly campaigning against smoking and alcohol.

The pill has become inextricably caught up in the heated public debate on modern morality which has flowed from the excesses of the so-called 'permissive society' but I feel that this constantly side-tracks the real issue at stake: women's health. The public debate is lively and entertaining, producing endless headlines and good TV documentaries. The conservatives blame liberals for creating a sexually irresponsible society and corrupting the young; the liberals counter by claiming that in not facing up to facts we are left to deal with the consequences of unwanted pregnancy. But morality has grown out of historical experience and it is now women and their children who will witness the disastrous effects of promiscuity on family life.

The issue of morality concerns me far less than the health of women, which is being sacrificed on the global altar of population control. In writing this book I am aware that there is a responsibility on me to point to other directions, to pill alternatives. Perhaps because steroid hormones have hogged the research picture for so long progress in other methods has been slow. But now older women are becoming aware of the problems associated with oral contraceptives and hormone therapy. They are also less happy about having an intra-uterine device inserted. An IUD has drawbacks which make it unsuitable for young women who are not yet ready to start their families.

IUDs

The exact mechanism of action of most IUDs (or coils) is not known. Possibilities suggested have been mechanical irritation or prostaglandin release preventing implantation. Copper IUDs change enzyme activities and may increase the number of pus cells which can destroy sperm. Copper, now sometimes covered in silver to slow down absorption, is toxic and high levels are found in the hair samples of users. Women who become pregnant with an IUD in place have a three times greater risk of a miscarriage and a ten times increased risk of an ectopic pregnancy — that is a pregnancy which embeds outside of the womb. IUD users have two and a half times the risk of pelvic inflammatory disease and infection of their tubes and endometrium that diaphragm or pill users have. As these infections can result in permanent infertility, they seem to be unwarranted risks for women who have not yet had children.

When IUDs first appeared on the contraceptive scene, I was highly sceptical of the wisdom of inserting a foreign body into such a highly reactive vascular area as the bed of the womb. Time has shown the method to be unsatisfactory for most women and the great majority stop using it within a few years — much the same result as the pill.

The Oxford/FPA study compared the risk of unplanned pregnancy with a wide range of contraceptive techniques.[1] The failure rate per 100 women-years for both male and female sterilisation was less than 0.1, while the risk with the combined oral contraceptive pills was between 0.14 and 0.44 depending on the doses used. The diaphragm at 2.4 was better than the progestogen-only pills at 3.0. With various types of IUDs, the risk ranged from 1.1 to 4.3 which, overall, compared favourably with the sheath at 4.3, although the risk with the sheath is probably less than this if chemical spermicides such as nonoxynol are always also used. Chemicals alone, without the use of a barrier method (either a diaphragm or a sheath), carried a risk of 14.8.

At admission to the study, diaphragm users were more likely to be long-term users — 52 per cent had used the diaphragm for more than five years, while only 12 per cent of pill users and 9 per cent of IUD users had persisted with their method for over five years.

IUD users were more likely, during the study, to be referred to hospital for anaemia, varicose veins, infected tubes (salpingitis) and were more likely to have cervical disease, dysplasia and carcinoma in situ, compared with diaphragm users. Attempts to improve the efficiency of the IUD so that the risks of pregnancy, expulsion, pain, infection and bleeding might be lessened, have resulted in chemicals being added. Slow release progesterone or progestogens are used to reduce the expulsion rate but they may increase irregular bleeding in sensitive women. To deal with this excessive blood loss antifibrinolytic and antiprostaglandin agents are being tested.

To provide sterilisation without surgery, it has been suggested that a chemical, such as quinacrine hydrochloride, can be carried by an IUD shape into the uterus where its release into the corners of the womb could theoretically block the fallopian tubes and provide sterilisation.

Barrier Methods

Barrier methods have been given a recent boost because of their protective value against some sexually transmitted diseases. These diseases have spread alarmingly since the fifties, with around 500,000 people in Britain going to STD clinics each year. Gonorrhea, genital herpes, non-specific urethritis and an infection called pelvic inflammatory disease (PID) have all been increased in the past two decades.

It was recently reported that women athletes, so aware of their physical health, have been turning away from the pill and using barrier methods. The research comes from the University of Illinois where 60 per cent of seventy female athletes surveyed preferred barrier methods of contraception, and only 13 per cent chose the pill.[2] Similar evidence comes from a study of women marathon runners.[3]

The much maligned sheath has been making a comeback with the blessing of the director of the Margaret Pyke Centre, Dr John Guillebaud. One of its advantages is that it protects both against gonorrhea and cervical cancer. It is thought to be favoured by first time users, is then relegated to second place by those in stable relationships, and returns to popularity for the middle-aged. One of the problems with the sheath has been the user. Pregnancies occur when it is not used properly and there have even been stories of husband or wife sabotage, with sheath breakage blamed for the resulting pregnancy. Sheaths which contain spermicide that helps to immobilise sperm are more effective but are also more expensive.

While the condom has been popular with men from all walks of life, the diaphragm has mostly been chosen by women in the higher social classes. Rubber diaphragms have been in use for about a hundred years and fit across the vault of the vagina covering the cervix. But, as the famous family planning pioneer, Dr Helena Wright used to say, 'They don't have to be glued in'. A diaphragm is designed to prevent sperm shooting directly into the womb and spermicide cream is used on its upper and lower surfaces to kill any sperm managing to swim round its rim.

For women who have poor muscle tone, or who are troubled by recurrent cystitis, different shapes and materials are available. The cervical cap fits the cervix by suction, while the vault cap or vimule may suit other women.

One of the objections to using a diaphragm is that it is messy because of the spermicidal cream, jelly or pessaries that are also necessary to ensure a low pregnancy risk. Because of this other types of cap have been developed. One, known as a honey cap because it is impregnated with honey, can be left in place for longer than the usually recommended twelve hours. Another American development is the Contracap which is now undergoing trials. A silicone mould is taken from each woman's cervix so that her cap can be worn continuously for several months as it has a one-way valve which allows menstrual blood and cervical secretions to be discharged downwards but prevents seminal fluid passing upwards.

An obvious drawback of these new methods is the chance of toxic-shock syndrome. Whether these cases are caused by the material in tampons or merely by obstruction of the cervical canal, is still debatable. For the same reason two new disposable and easily inserted sponges being tested have also raised doubts and seem much less reliable. Another possible complication of female barrier methods is endometriosis, which may be encouraged by retrograde blood flow from the uterus along the fallopian tubes. My own preference is for a diaphragm used in the traditional way.

Natural Family Planning

Along with many others, doctors and lay people alike, I have been concerned about the effectiveness of natural family planning. It sounds so wonderful, with the woman and her partner managing to space their family without recourse to

190

drugs or invasive techniques, but the track record is not good. Dr Anna Flynn, an expert in natural contraception, quotes an old joke which runs 'What do you call people who use the rhythm method of birth control?' The reply is — 'parents'.

But the techniques for identifying the exact time of maximum fertility are becoming more precise and should lead to simpler ways for women to spot the times in their cycle when lovemaking is likely to result in a pregnancy. One of the simplest ideas yet is being developed in the laboratory. This is a 'dipstick' which can pick up the change in the level of oestrogen excreted in the urine. When the fertile time occurs, the dipstick will change colour. It may be several years before such a unique development comes to our help, so in the meantime, what is available in non-toxic contraception?

Natural family planning is a technique which has to be learned. There are several ways for a woman to learn of her fertile phase, by temperature check, or identification of the stages of mucus, or by the condition of the cervix. The best known proponent of natural methods is Dr Flynn, a research fellow in gynaecology at Birmingham Maternity Hospital, and a founder of the National Association of Natural Family Planning Teachers (NANFPT) who runs orientation courses for doctors to learn the latest methods.[4] Full courses last six months and the doctors are trained to teach natural family planning and fertility awareness. Some GPs who have taken this training have set up clinics in their health centres where patients can be referred if they wish, but this is a very new development.

Since the thirties doctors have been able to teach women to recognise certain symptoms of the fertile phase but most methods involved taking early morning temperatures until the Billings[5] ovulation method used cervical mucus as a guide. Now women can be taught a whole range of signs, including mood changes, for additional help in detecting the fertile phase.

We used to guess that the egg survived for two to three days after ovulation, and the sperm for a few days. We now know that the egg only has a life of between 12 and 24 hours whereas the sperm can survive for up to six days. As pregnancy can only occur during the day that the egg is living it would seem that the perfect method of birth control would be to identify this one particular day, but the picture is complicated by the fact that the sperm can be 'stored' and swim out to meet an egg on the day it is released.

Women are taught to identify the types of mucus to tell them where they are in the cycle. After the period there is no mucus and this is the early pre-ovulatory infertile phase. As the egg grows the increasing oestrogen causes mucus to be secreted and the fertile phase begins. From this time on the mucus increases in amount and looks different. There is a lot of watery, almost transparent mucus which reaches a peak when the egg is released, and on the day this happens a woman is most fertile. I have heard the mucus of the fertile pre-ovulatory period aptly described as 'motorway mucus' because under the microscope it has clear, straight lanes which attract sperm to zip along!

The mucus changes in appearance by the drop in oestrogen and the presence of progesterone once the egg is released, and it becomes a sticky plug. This mucus is an impediment to sperm and the less fertile phase begins. However Dr Flynn teaches that 36 hours must be allowed for ovulation and 24 hours for the egg to survive. The post-ovulatory infertile phase starts in earnest three days after what she calls 'maximum mucus grading' (MMG) and lasts for ten to twelve days until the next menstrual period.

By itself, the ovulation method is unsatisfactory, because other factors enter the picture and there are variations in each woman and each cycle which may lengthen or shorten the fertile phase. And sometimes 'fertile' mucus can appear on supposedly non-fertile days and confuse a woman.

The daily temperature-taking method has improved with the marketing of electronic thermometers which give a reading within a few seconds. The thermometers have specially wide gradings, necessary for a woman to notice the small change in temperature which indicates that ovulation has taken place and the rest of the cycle will be infertile. The body's temperature is low in the first half of a cycle and rises in the second, either quickly or in steps, and women are taught to recognise this. Once the reading is high for three consecutive days you are entering a 'safe' zone. The temperature will stay high until the next period. In the case of pregnancy, the temperature stays up for about twenty days after ovulation — one of the first signs. But even here a double check is prudent. The temperature change by itself does not give enough warning of fertile days before ovulation. Sperm can still reach the uterus in mucus and lie in wait for ovulation.

The sympto-thermal method combines several signs to identify safe periods — a check on every possible sign the body gives. Particularly useful is to check the condition of the cervix by finger. In the non-fertile part of the cycle it is low, dry and firm, as contrasted with the wet, soft sensation caused by the rise in oestrogen in the fertile phase.

A study of the ovulation method was organised by a World Health Organisation task force in 1977 involving 725 women in New Zealand, Ireland, the Philippines, San Salvador and India.[6] The results were published in December 1983 showing an overall failure rate of 2 per cent, with probable conception in the non-fertile phase put at 0.4 per cent.

It was shown that there was a 50 per cent pregnancy risk if couples made love during the three to one days before ovulation when the sticky 'plug' mucus was produced. If intercourse took place at the same time but in the presence of watery mucus, the risk increased to 54 per cent. But on each day following the peak ovulation day, the risk decreased, down to 9 per cent on the third day.

But however effective these methods are they are only suitable for highly motivated couples who already have a secure, stable, loving relationship in which sharing problems is possible. Apart from the motivation needed to learn the techniques and apply them with concentration, couples may have to abstain from intercourse for up to fourteen days — five days of menstruation plus up to nine days during the fertile phases. And factors such as emotional upsets, flying abroad and illness may cause a woman's ovulation to be disrupted.

For the average non-motivated person, or for the adolescent who goes along to family planning clinics, these methods are still too complicated. It will need much more research to find one extremely simple technique which can either identify safe days *absolutely* for the years before a family is wanted, or after one has been completed.

New Developments

Contraception for Men

What of better contraception for men? What research is being carried out into this area now that women are voicing their reluctance to be held solely responsible for family planning? It is depressing to find that research is still fixed into the exogenous hormone scene, with the World Health Organisation backing the development of oral or injectable drugs.

I can hardly condemn the use of synthetic hormones in contraception for women and condone their use in men! For either sex I think they are disastrous, and this is why we have not seen their speedier appearance as male contraceptives. In earlier research it was discovered that men could not drink alcohol while on their 'pill' and that was an immediate setback. The more pressing problem for the scientists however is to produce a drug which inhibits fertility without interfering with sex drive. Of course, sex drive was one of the casualties of many women on the pill. In the early sixties Dr Margaret Jackson reported that her (Devon) women patients even thought that was how the pill worked, by cutting out the desire for sex. It seems that this is one side-effect which pill scientists have deemed acceptable for women, but not for men.

The problems of producing a drug for men with minimal side-effects appears to have dampened enthusiasm in the pharmaceutical industry. Professor S. L. Jeffcoate of the Chelsea Hospital for Women has reported a noticeable lack of interest among the drug companies.[7] He cites the lack of knowledge of male fertility as an obstacle, but a similar lack of knowledge of female reproduction does not appear to have halted production of the pill.

Trials with a synthetic analogue of testosterone have not come to much because of side-effects — weight gain, breast enlargement and a slight decrease in libido. Potency in men is also hit by the use of oestrogens, which have been shown to reduce sperm counts to sub-fertile. Testicular size is also affected, so oestrogens do not have potential for male contraception. There are however WHO backed trials currently looking at a progestogen-androgen preparation. As in women, progestogens will produce reversible fertility in men. On their own progestogens cut down sex drive so an androgen is added to make up for the lack of endogenous androgen production and to restore potency. Sperm counts have been shown to be reduced on certain doses of this compound.[8] Should hormonal contraception ever take off for men, I would expect to see similar health problems appearing in them as I have outlined in women.

Sterilization

There was some talk of a reversible sterilization technique, such as a clip, at a clinical ecology conference I attended in 1979, but not much seems to have come of this. There would be problems, however, for such a device must not damage the highly delicate tubes. It is easier to gum up the tubes than to unstick them again.

Research continues in finding different ways of administering hormones, by implants, IUD, sponge cap, vaccines and sprays, but these are really 'old steroids with new uses' and I cannot see that they represent progress. A recently described ring containing a progestogen ensures that the steroid is as near the cervix as possible. So far, the main alternatives to the pill are effective barrier methods, natural family planning and male and female sterilization. These last two have suffered some unfortunate adverse publicity although for couples who have completed their families and are unable or unwilling to use barrier methods, vasectomy or female sterilization is a good choice. For younger couples, however, who may want further children later it is of course useless and it is no good at all for the single young.

Most of our pill trial volunteers of the sixties were married women who had all the children they wanted, and many opted for sterilization when they developed serious pill side-effects. In spite of claims to the contrary, controlled studies show women are not more likely to become depressed after sterilization and some report improved sexual satisfaction[9] probably because their libido returned after stopping the pill and because they were freed from the anxiety of further pregnancies. Sterilization is now the method most commonly used by married couples.

When it was found that vasectomised monkeys had sperm antibodies and an increased risk of atherosclerosis, it was feared that the operation would render men more susceptible to heart attacks, strokes and hypertension. This has made men nervous of the procedure. But two recent reports, from the Radcliffe Infirmary and Yale University Medical School, indicate that the operation does not increase the risk of heart disease. More long-term studies are needed, however, as few men over fifty-five, in the UK at least, have had vasectomies.[10]

Still at an early stage of development is a vaccination against pregnancy. It is estimated that about 5 per cent of infertile women may have antibodies circulating in their blood which prevent conception. Antizona antibodies block the attachment of sperm to the zona pellucida which surrounds the ovum.

Another type of vaccine to hCG, the hormone produced by the embryo, has been suggested but this hormone is chemically similar to the mother's own pituitary hormones.

Immunology, although a rapidly advancing field of medicine, is still in its infancy, and after our experience with the pill women have every reason to be cautious.

What Should We Say To The Young?

When the pill became available my father-in-law, minister of a Scottish cathedral, said it would cause widespread promiscuity. In those days I was still delighted with the pill's 100 per cent efficiency and I naively believed that we would be able to handle this new freedom responsibly. But no, he was right. Girls are freely given the pill — a passport to sexual licence — at younger and younger ages even though it is illegal for a man to have sexual intercourse with a girl under sixteen. Some people think more counselling is needed. What does that mean? Which girl, keen to sleep with a boyfriend to prevent him going off with someone else, is going to be persuaded that she should wait for a few years and miss the 'fun' her friends are having?

Contrary to popular opinion, the pill has not prevented abortions. The termination rate for the under twenties doubled between the late sixties and the early seventies and has risen from 8.9 per 1,000 unmarried women in 1969 to 22.5 in 1981. It has been estimated that in 1970 only 9 per cent of single women in England and Wales aged sixteen to thirty-five had ever taken the pill. Now the main group of first time users are schoolgirls or students, and as doctors were able to prescribe the pill for underage girls without informing their parents the age of first pill use is still falling. Abortion rates are rising again with this latest increase in early sexual activity. But for schoolgirls the pill may seem safer than it really is. They are likely to be at their most healthy, doing regular exercise, and able to tolerate the pill without obvious side-effects. But are they mortgaging their future and their chances of having normal healthy families? Because they are starting the pill so much younger the gap between them stopping it, either for side-effects or because they are ready to become pregnant, is likely to be that much longer. Once they stop the pill they will need to use alternative methods which require self discipline and co-operation with a reliable partner and it is likely that the abortion rate will increase because as yet no other form of contraceptive is as reliable.

The pill, in a big enough dose, is the only method of contraception that can guarantee complete and usually reversible sterility. It is the only method truly suited to 'safe' sex. But what else is it doing? It is blocking brain hormones and acting on young ovaries. It is changing metabolism at a critical time of growth, sexual and emotional development. Human beings are not fully mature at puberty but go on changing until the end of their early twenties. The first, often irregular, periods do not mean a girl has become a woman.

If the pill is too dangerous for a woman to use it is clearly much too dangerous for children. We are assaulting our future genetic pool. At a time of falling intellectual and behavioural standards of our children, there is no room for complacency. No wonder doctors were advised not to break a girl's confidentiality and tell the parents. Her mother is likely to be only too well aware of the pill's side-effects. She has probably already had first hand experience.

It has been part of human culture throughout history to protect our future — our young women. Customs and habits have prized virginity. Women's wonderfully evolved and complicated bodies are too easily permanently damaged. Fallopian tubes are too quickly blocked. We must protect our innocent young before it is too late for them to learn to protect themselves.

Intellectuals as diverse as Valerie Riches and Germaine

Greer are now united in their advice to the young. A Responsible Society pamphlet advises 'Saying No'[11] while the book *Sex and Destiny*[12] warns 'avoid intromission'. It may seem strange to imagine a society where young people wait until they are older until they start having sex but this was the normal state of affairs before the pill. There were very few abortions carried out among the very young. If the pill was banned, there may be an increase in unwanted pregnancies but it is hoped that social customs could quickly change. An example of this has been the fall in numbers attending STD clinics in America because of the AIDS scare.

Some women say the pill gives them control over their lives. They do not have to trust men to take precautions. But taking the pill does not give women control over their health. On the contrary, a woman taking hormones can never be sure which illness will next appear. Individual men may not reliably always use withdrawal (coitus interruptus or the Roman method), or always use sheaths and chemicals, but the great reduction in family size from the six to ten children common in the Victorian age throughout Europe, to an average of two children has been largely brought about by men responsibly making the decision before clinics for women were generally available. Surely the very act of sexual intercourse is one of mutual trust. If a woman cannot trust the man, she should not be having such a relationship.

Countries, like Russia, who have never allowed the pill, have a very high abortion rate and this is a cause for great concern. Abortions increase the risk of infertility and physical and emotional problems. However, my experience is that, with the majority of older responsible couples, barrier methods especially the diaphragm and spermicides are usually extremely effective and can be used for most of a woman's fertile life. When I advise a woman to stop taking the pill and fit a cap, her usual reaction is to be pleasantly surprised that it is less trouble than she expected. Spermicides carry a slightly increased risk of fetal abnormalities if they are used during the month conception takes place but not if they have only been used in the preceding month. A combination of barrier and natural methods may be ideal for many couples.

The commonest method used in modern times, before the pill, to restrict population and family size was withdrawal. Again, this can be a highly effective method for couples who have found it works for them. Family size has remained below replacement level of 2.5 in this country since the 1920s and means it is the average family size which is the main controlling factor of population growth. In China the population problem is so serious that only one child per family is allowed. Small families mean we want healthy children. Steroids increase the chances of damaged babies; it is time to say no to the pill.

The story of the pill is not just one of dark political intrigue or even of merely huge financial profits. It is not any one story. It is the scandal of collusion on a massive world wide scale. Women want to take the pill. Men want women to be always available. It is human nature to want something for nothing. Contraception with no risk of pregnancy for the first time in human history.

A mother with a brain haemorrhage wanted to continue taking the pill; unmarried women, as Germaine Greer has described, denied their side-effects. Mothers and even fathers, fearful in a permissive age, want their young daughters to go on the pill. Sadly, scientist doctors, who find they are unable to continue with depressing pill research give up, when their humanity is greatly needed. Many other reasons are found for the appalling increase in ill health among the young. We are all to blame — but the evidence is that the real victim is the future generation. The time for clear vision is long overdue.

So what has been the cost?

It took ten to fifteen years to synthesise the first pills from natural hormones. As our knowledge of side-effects has increased, so developmental research has become more sophisticated and it can now take up to twenty or thirty years to market a new product, a commitment few large companies are keen to undertake even though they have been paid very large sums of money by the British tax payer. In the seventies up to three and a half million women were given free pills by the NHS each year. The trade price of similar pills varies according to market competition from between 23p and £1.15 but at the height of the pill's popularity the average cost of commonly used pills was about £1. This means that the Government was paying out roughly £50m each year to buy hormone contraceptive pills for British women, not counting what was spent on pills for women in under-developed countries as part of overseas aid and on hormones for other purposes which are a great deal more expensive. Although there has been a decrease since the seventies in the number of women taking the pill, there are still just under three million who do. The real cost, however, has been much greater. It is impossible to estimate what has been spent 'papering over the cracks' treating or alleviating the illness, social tragedies and handicaps that have been caused by the pill. No British government would now hand out free cigarettes and yet the pill causes as much illness as smoking.

So far the search for alternative contraceptives has concentrated on new steroid hormones, better barrier methods, immunological techniques and improving fertility awareness. Steroids affect the whole body, immunological methods may not be reversible, while barrier methods seem to be a return to the past.

Dr Hugh Cox, now running a highly cost-effective NHS practice as a clinical ecologist, was Director of Clinical Research in the sixties with the company which made the only all-British pill. Since he studied the changes caused by the steroid pills with me he has been thinking about alternatives. At a very basic level we are all made up of positive and negative electrical charges and he believes it might be possible to make use of this — perhaps by reversing the normal tiny potential across the cervix when a woman is in the fertile part of her cycle. Feasible or not, new ideas need to be investigated in research institutes dedicated to reproductive physiology and staffed by scientists and doctors of the highest calibre to make sure, if possible, that we do not repeat our mistakes. Vested interests and personal prejudices should not obscure facts. We have interfered with our bodies' most critical, delicate and sensitive mechanisms and have launched what Germaine Greer has named 'The Dark Age of Steroids'.

The search for a safe contraceptive is of great priority, so that we can regulate our fertility sanely and responsibly. Because of the pill we have become accustomed to a method of contraception that is both reliable and convenient. People's expectations have risen accordingly and when we seek an alternative it must be one that has the pill's benefits but not its side-effects, particularly if we are to help the third world countries. So far our interference with cultures and traditions may have caused more problems than it has solved, but we have to go on trying. Our aim must be to find a contraceptive which will not permanently damage ovaries, sperm or testes, or have any systemic effect. Women, children and families should not be sacrificed to the god of perfect contraception.

APPENDIX I
Body Chemistry and Nutrition

Normal Adrenal Hormones

The pituitary gland lies at the base of the brain, behind the eyes. It is divided into two parts. The front (anterior) part secretes hormones which affect growth, thyroid activity, sexual function, lactation and water, carbohydrate, protein and fat metabolism by regulating the secretions of the other endocrine glands. The hormones in the posterior part of the pituitary control the conservation of the body's water by the kidneys and cause the womb to contract during labour at the end of pregnancy.

When Dr Raymond Greene described the premenstrual syndrome with Dr Dalton in 1953[1], they knew that progesterone relieved the symptoms of some women. Dr Greene, however, remained doubtful that progesterone therapy was a universal panacea. He thought the hypothesis was too facile and felt that few disorders in endocrinology were so simply explained. He emphasised that water retention, such an important part of the syndrome, was a sign of adrenal hormone overactivity.

All steroid hormones are close chemical relatives, sharing a similar four ring structure. They are made from a fatty substance, cholesterol, which is manufactured in the liver, stored and concentrated in the gall bladder before being released with the bile into the gut. Cholesterol is also made in the ovaries, testes, or the two adrenal glands where it is converted into a variety of steroid hormones.

The small adrenals lie above each kidney and the vascular middle part of the gland secretes hormones like adrenaline which give us our instant 'fight or flight' reactions. These hormones are related to proteins and do not have a steroid structure but the outer layer of the adrenal, called the cortex, makes over forty different steroid hormones, usually classified in three main groups according to how they regulate cell metabolism.

1. The Androgens
2. The Glucocorticoids
3. The Mineral-Corticoids

The Androgens

The adrenal male sex hormones, mostly testosterone, retain nitrogen and help to build up the body's muscles and protein — known as an anabolic effect. Anabolic steroids are the subject of controversy in sport where they are used by some competitors to stimulate muscle strength and endurance. These hormones were probably originally designed to promote cell growth and later, during evolution, became geared to regulate bisexual reproduction. Anabolic hormones stimulate metabolism and form sugars and proteins inside cells. This leads to vigorous cell and blood vessel growth. The cell walls become flexible allowing easy transport of metabolites.

The adrenals of both men and women make small amounts of oestrogens and progesterone. Although most of a woman's female hormone production is from the ovary, after the menopause the adrenals become her main source of oestrogen. Men have high blood levels of testosterone, made in the testes and adrenals, but women convert only small amounts of their adrenal androgens into active testosterone. In both sexes growth is also controlled by many other regulators including the pituitary's growth hormone and thyroid hormones.

The Glucocorticoids

These are released during stress and temporarily stop cell metabolism, known as a catabolic effect. The main hormone cortisol blocks insulin secretion and raises blood sugar levels by changing the protein building blocks (amino acids) into sugar (glucose) which is stored in the liver. Catabolic hormones also make the cell walls rigid and less permeable to ions, like sodium and potassium, passing in and out of the cells. As this is how nerve impulses are transmitted, large doses of cortisone or prednisone can cause emotional imbalance, irritability and depression and even a schizophrenia-like psychosis or temporary madness. Everyone can suffer from stress if it is prolonged and severe enough — as was discovered in the trenches during the First World War.

Catabolic steroids also suppress the inflammatory reactions which are the body's response to injury, infection or immune changes. They have been widely used to give temporary relief for illnesses like asthma and arthritis but their side-effects can be disastrous, including high blood pressure, changes in fat and water metabolism, with obesity and a round 'moon' face and thin bones — osteoporosis, by interfering with bone cell metabolism. They can also cause sticky platelets and senile osteoporosis can be caused by masses of small thrombi forming in the bones. Patients taking steroids have an increased susceptibility to infection and are less able to deal with carcinogens because of changes in liver function.

In her book *Bone Behaviour*[2] Dr Kitty Little writes 'the hormone balance may approach the catabolic [stopping growth] during the later stages of pregnancy and after childbirth, after the menopause, during old age, when corticosteroids are given for therapeutic purposes, or as a result of oral contraceptive agents. A combination of factors may result in corticosteroid levels exceeding the threshold for thrombus formation. This threshold depends on other chemicals affecting the pituitary-adrenal system. It is abnormally low for contraceptive agents.' In animal experiments, Dr Little found the male hormone testosterone had a greater effect on cell and blood vessel growth than the normal female hormones. But she discovered that the synthetic progestogen derivatives of testosterone caused more overgrowth of blood vessels than testosterone with one progestogen causing more changes than another.

Mineral-Corticoids

The main hormone controlling salt and water metabolism is aldosterone, which instructs the kidneys to retain sodium and excrete potassium. This can result in such a rapid rise in blood pressure that aldosterone is never given to patients. These mineral-corticoids are regulated by a kidney-blood vessel system involving renin and angiotensin. One of the reasons oral contraceptives cause high blood pressure is because they can increase the blood renin activity.

The other adrenal steroids are controlled by the brain via the hypothalamus and the secretion of ACTH (adreno cortico trophic hormone) from the pituitary. In turn, ACTH secretion is blocked by high levels of cortisol or sex hormones as part of a negative feed-back system. It is also altered by the body's daily clock, or diurnal rhythm, which is why we tend to feel better at some times of the day than others, but normally the most powerful, overriding mechanism is stress. Stress includes injury, pain, fear, worry, nausea, fever, low blood sugar, and especially jealousy.

The fact that the high levels of sex hormones can switch off ACTH means that the very powerful pill hormones can easily interfere with the body's stress coping mechanisms at the same time as they are blocking the ovulation stimulating hormones.

The problem is that steroid hormones have the same basic structure with many overlapping effects so that when a woman's hormone levels change they set off many other changes in their metabolism. Nature developed the sex hormones to be fairly specific but when man altered them in the laboratory so that they worked by mouth, they became more powerful — and primitive. The pill progestogens can be oestrogenic, antioestrogenic, androgenic as well as progestogenic. Pill hormones are water soluble and excreted in the urine but natural hormones are fat soluble and become stored in body fats of animals or women treated with these hormones.

Changes in the Pill

Most of the work on pill metabolism in the UK has been carried out by Professor Victor Wynn and his team at the metabolic unit, St Mary's Hospital, Paddington. He was already investigating anabolic steroids in the 1950s and had discovered that the oral synthetic hormones were more likely to alter liver function, fat and carbohydrate metabolism than the original natural parent hormones. Professor Wynn speculated that as the oral progestogens were very similar to synthetic anabolic steroids they might also cause widespread upsets.

There was another reason Professor Wynn expected oestrogens and progestogens to cause diabetes. They were being used to mimic pregnancy — and when some women are pregnant the blood sugar (glucose) tends to rise and spill out into the urine.

Carbohydrate Metabolism

In 1966 the St Mary's team published findings showing that nearly one in five women taking different oral contraceptives mostly with mestranol 0.1mg, had abnormally high glucose levels and one woman developed exceptionally high values.[3] Since then Professor Wynn has seen maturity-onset diabetes caused by the pill in a number of patients.

Microdosage Pill

In 1982 Professor Wynn published his study on the lowest dose pill then available.[4] Three years before, he had given 210 healthy young women, mostly aged between twenty-five and thirty, the lowest dose combined pill then on the market — 150 micrograms levonorgestrel and 30 micrograms ethinyl oestradiol. After fifteen months, 60 per cent of the women had stopped taking it and after three years only 8 per cent were still using it, 42 per cent having been lost to follow-up. Only 10 per cent were known to have stopped because they no longer required contraceptives.

Of the thirty-nine women who started their third year, two (5 per cent) developed deep vein thrombosis and another woman had superficial venous thrombosis. Four had a sustained rise in blood pressure after one year of use, which reverted to normal when they stopped the pill, and one woman developed an abnormal electrocardiogram. Six women developed abnormal glucose tolerance tests and some of the women deteriorated into the diabetic range with continued treatment, improving when they stopped. One woman made this jump twice. Just over one quarter stopped the pill for 'minor' side-effects — weight gain, headache, depression, diminished libido, breakthrough bleeding, amenorrhoea and nausea — while another 11 per cent asked for a change of pill.

Progressive Deterioration

During this study, even the women who seemed well had a progressive deterioration in their glucose tolerance. This means a woman's metabolism becomes more abnormal the longer she takes the pill, whether she has symptoms or not. The insulin secretion rose at first but eventually did not keep up with the rising glucose values. Professor Wynn's conclusion was that this combination of steroids was too strong for contraceptive use and he suggested a weaker, less androgenic progestogen such as norethindrone should be used, but Dr Little had noticed this was likely to distort blood vessels.

Since 1970 it has been known that injections of large amounts of progesterone (300 to 400mg per day), which is similar in amount to the endogenous progesterone secretion in the latter third of pregnancy, causes changes in carbohydrate metabolism. The glucose tolerance is impaired, as in diabetes, and there is an increased resistance to insulin — injections of insulin are less likely to lower the blood sugar. Professor William Spellacy's group in Chicago worked out that oral microdoses of a progestogen with male hormone-like actions, given as oral contraceptives, can alter carbohydrate metabolism as much as these large doses of progesterone given by injection. From the doses used it can be worked out that megestrol acetate, norethisterone and ethynodiol diacetate are roughly a thousand times and norgestrel five thousand times more powerful than progestogen in this effect.[5] The chance of the pill causing diabetes is increased by its male hormone like actions but is also increased by the oestrogen which is added to most pills. Oral androgens, anabolic steroids and danazol, used to suppress breast lumps, can have similar adverse effects on glucose tolerance and are particularly antagonistic to insulin.

Fat Metabolism

In his 1966 studies, Professor Wynn had also discovered that the current combined pills raised the levels of blood fats: cholesterol, triglycerides and nonesterified free fatty acids.[6] The most striking change was a raised blood pyruvate which is known to happen if glucocorticoid adrenal hormones like hydrocortisone are given. Professor Wynn's later studies have shown that the higher the dose or balance of oestrogens, which increase the effect of the body's cortisol, the greater is the increase in the blood fats.

This was quite puzzling as young men have more heart attacks than young women. After the menopause the blood fat levels in women become more like those in men and post menopausal women have nearly the same risk of heart attack as men.

For years the increased risk of arterial disease was thought to be linked to blood cholesterol levels which also increase with age, but it is now thought that heart attack risk relates to *lowered* levels of a fraction of cholesterol called HDL_2 (high density lipoprotein). The lower the HDL_2 level, the greater seems to be the risk of hardening of the arteries, atherosclerosis.

In 1982 Professor Wynn reported that, out of a group of low dose pills, the more androgenic pills lowered the HDL_2 values more than the oestrogenic pills. As little as 35 micrograms of norgestrel or 350 micrograms of norethisterone given alone as a progestogen-only pill significantly lowered the HDL_2[7] levels. This means the increased risk of heart attacks did relate to the androgen induced fat changes. When a small amount of oestrogen, 30 micrograms of ethinyl oestradiol, was added to 150 micrograms norgestrel, the HDL_2 levels remained lower and there were also significant triglyceride and carbohydrate alterations.

Professor Wynn's predictions have been correct. Contraceptive pills cause similar metabolic changes to anabolic steroids but the changes are also like pregnancy when extra cortisol is secreted giving an effect of prolonged stress.

Gall bladder disease is twice as likely with higher dose oestrogen pills — seven in 1,000 women observed in the RCGP study — because of raised cholesterol and blood fats such as triglycerides, but the progestogen MPA has been found to significally stop gall bladder emptying, increasing gall stone formation.[8]

Liver Function

We now know that alterations to enzyme activity in the liver — the body's metabolic factory — are crucial in causing women on the pill to become more and more allergic or reactive to increasing numbers of foods and chemicals. Mostly, progestogens tend to slow liver clearance. Normally men and older people have slower rates of clearance than young women. Smoking and tea and coffee speed up liver clearance. Several drugs, including medicines used to treat tuberculosis and epilepsy, alter liver clearance and increase the risks of pregnancy especially with low dose pills.[9] Patients taking oestrogens are more likely to develop toxic side-effects with the tricyclic antidepressant drug imipramine as oestrogens block the drug's metabolism. (See page 52.)

Broad spectrum antibiotics like ampicillin and neomycin may interfere with the gut-liver circulation of steroids, probably because they kill off gut bacteria, and pregnancies and irregular bleeding have been reported. This is important as women taking the pill have a greater chance of developing infections.

If vitamin C is given with ethinyl oestradiol, the two drugs compete to be excreted by the gut wall. If 1gm of ascorbic acid is given, the plasma levels of the oestrogen increase by 50 per cent which effectively can turn a low dose oestrogen pill into a high dose pill, above the limit set by the Committee for Safety of Medicines in 1969. But vitamin C is required for the body's cleansing antioxidant mechanisms which are under strain among pill users.

Protein Metabolism

Proteins are made up of separate essential building blocks called amino acids. Cheese, especially mouldy cheese, has large amounts of tyramine, while chocolate contains a lot of phenylethylamine. Amines help to transmit nerve impulses

211

so they are involved in the control of mood and behaviour. The same chemicals also change blood vessel reactions. Eating cheese or chocolate can make you feel good but if you eat too much you can get a migraine.

The pill switches around protein and amine metabolism. Proteins are broken down in the liver by two main pathways — the tryptophan-serotonin pathway and the dopamine adrenaline pathway. Tryptophan is carried in the blood, bound to plasma proteins which are increased by oestrogens and lowered by anabolic hormones like progestogen and androgens which encourage protein breakdown.

Serotonin

In the sixties abnormally high levels of serotonin and its end products were discovered during migraine attacks. At the same time it was discovered that brains of suicide victims had too little serotonin.

Serotonin is made from tryptophan which is also too low in clinically depressed patients. As oestrogens increase the levels of plasma proteins they release more tryptophan into the blood stream and have been used to treat depression. But synthetic oestrogens and the combined pill raise cortisol levels which increases the enzymatic breakdown of tryptophan in the liver and can cause a shortage of serotonin. Unfortunately the breakdown is carried out by an abnormal pathway and in 1966 Dr David Rose, working at St Mary's with Professor Wynn, found that all pill users therefore had abnormal end products of metabolism in their urine.[10] These metabolites are carcinogenic and can cause bladder cancer.

As pill users have less tryptophan available to make serotonin they are more likely to be depressed. Large amounts of vitamin B_6 — pyridoxine — are used up in this increased tryptophan secretion and Dr Adams found 40 per cent of women had evidence of tissue deficiency in this vitamin.[11] Vitamin B_6 taken with the pill may help prevent depression but the abnormal metabolism starts further back in the pathway and there are many other abnormalities. Zinc also becomes deficient.

Adams found that when the B_6 deficient women were given extra B_6 there was an improvement in their carbohydrate metabolism and they had fewer abnormal metabolites. But Professor Wynn discovered that glucose tolerance deteriorates with length of time taking the pill, so it is unlikely that B_6 or zinc supplementation would go on helping indefinitely. All pill users produce abnormal metabolites whether they are vitamin deficient or not. Pyridoxine did not improve glucose tolerance in the 60 per cent of women with normal vitamin B_6 levels. Extra vitamin B_6 only improved pill-induced depression in the women with measureable B_6 deficiency and had no effect on the others.[12]

Adrenaline

B_6 is also required for normal adrenaline metabolism. Oestrogens and combined pills lower blood tyrosine levels. Again the normal metabolism is diverted from making dopamine, noradrenaline and adrenaline to an abnormal pathway.[13]

MAO (monoamine oxidase)

Both serotonin and adrenaline are inactivated by the enzyme MAO. We know that progestogenic pills have high MAO activity and oestrogen pills low MAO activity in the endometrium. If the brain amines follow suit, it is easy to see why some women have migraine (high amines), some depression (low amines), and some, both, as the amine levels fluctuate above and below the normal range.

COMT (Catechol-o-methyl transferase)

Another enzyme which mops up and inactivates adrenaline when it's no longer required is COMT. At the Royal Surrey

County Hospital, Guildford and Surrey University, we measured red blood cell levels of COMT. Most women with migraine had levels within the normal range. But some women taking the same pill had too high or too low levels of COMT activity. Nearly all the women who were taking ergotamine every day to prevent a migraine attack (ergotamine addicts) had abnormal levels.[14,15]

Trace Mineral Metabolism

Most of the body's enzymes need small amounts of trace metals such as iron, zinc and copper to act like some vitamins as co-enzymes or catalysts in reactions. Again, like vitamins, too much or too little can be harmful. If there is a shortage of a key trace metal, an alternative metal may be substituted which means enzyme activity can increase or decrease.

(Figures show approximate mineral content of food in milligrams per 100 grams edible portion as published by Mineralab.)

Copper

Oysters 13.7   Brazil Nuts 2.3   Soy Lecithin 2.1
Almonds 1.4

Both MAO and COMT are copper containing enzymes. The biggest change in trace metals caused by the pill happens to copper. In 1968, Halsted, Hackly and Smith found that women taking the pill had blood copper levels more than twice as high as normal and much higher than in pregnancy. Women, who were aware of having side-effects had three times as much copper.[16]

Oestrogen and combined pills raise blood protein levels and copper is bound to a protein — ceruloplasmin. Even doses as low as 30 micrograms of ethinyl oestradiol double ceruloplasmin levels, a rise which is not decreased in combined pills.[17] This can make the plasma blue-green in colour which has worried blood bankers on occasion. Smoking also raises blood copper and ceruloplasmin, so a woman who both smokes and takes the pill is likely to have far too much copper. These high toxic levels of copper can be monitored by hair tests. Dr Elizabeth Lodge Rees, an American paediatrician who has great experience of using hair tests in clinical practice, always suspects oestrogen or pill use when a hair sample has a very high copper level. Copper IUDs can also elevate hair copper but usually not to such a great an extent as the pill.

Copper and zinc are antagonistic to each other and the correct copper to zinc ratio is essential for normal enzyme function. When we investigated liver function by using the antipyrine clearance test, we measured plasma copper and zinc at the same time. The normal copper zinc ratio was 1.0 to 1.7. Migraine patients with abnormal liver function had significantly higher ratios. The highest value 5 belonged to a laboratory worker who was at first investigated as a control but she also had migraine and was smoking and taking the pill.

In 1972 Pfeiffer and Iliev discovered that some schizophrenics taking the pill had exceptionally high blood copper levels.[18] The normal 0.9—1.2 micrograms/ml rises to 2.2 micrograms/ml by the end of pregnancy but some schizophrenics taking the pill had values of 2.6 to 5.65 micrograms/ml.

Professor Pfeiffer and others link high copper to high blood pressure and heart attacks, post-partum depression and pychosis and pre-eclampsia in pregnancy.

Zinc

Oysters 149   Ginger 7   Red Meat 5.5   Nuts 4

Zinc is one of the most important trace metals. It is necessary for the normal functioning of more than ninety enzymes including acid and alkaline phosphates. It is essential for normal cell division, protein synthesis and growth. The stability of both DNA and RNA requires the presence of bound zinc, which means zinc deficiency can induce chromosome abnormalities.

The pill reduces zinc levels. Adults need 15mg of zinc each day and pregnant women much more. Many modern diets have between 8 to 11mg per day, and zinc deficiency has become commonplace. It can be suspected if a person has white spots on their nails, a poor sense of taste and hair loss. Pregnant and lactating women may have tissue levels 33 per cent below normal. Zinc is lowered more with oestrogen alone than with the combined pill. Zinc deficiency is especially likely to cause immune upsets increasing the chance of allergies and infections. If a woman is zinc deficient at the start of her pregnancy she may be more likely to have an abnormal baby or a child with learning defects or hyperactivity. Smoking also causes zinc deficiency. Zinc deficiency may also cause localised damage to blood vessels. Women with anorexia, diabetes, schizophrenia and depression; children with learning difficulties and hyperactivity and cancer patients are all likely to be short of zinc.

Iron

Kelp 100   Yeast 17   Wheat bran 15   Liver 9

Most combined pills have strongly progestogenic action on the lining of the womb which becomes very thin. Withdrawal bleeding tends to be very scanty. Although the hemoglobin levels usually remain the same, serum iron increases in pill users possibly due to mobilization from bone marrow stores. A few pill users develop heavy irregular bleeding and more develop fibroids than non-pill users. The Walnut Creek study of 1981 reported significantly more women had severe iron deficiency anaemia needing hospital admission if they had ever used the pill or oestrogens.

Magnesium

Kelp 760   Wheat bran 490   Almonds 270   Cashews 267

Magnesium is a co-factor in 200 enzymes. Sweat analysis has shown that magnesium deficiency is second only to zinc deficiency in frequency. It is lowered by oestrogens and progestogens and, depending on the hormone balance and individual susceptibility, some women have magnesium deficiency with the pill. This can raise aldosterone levels and increase the chance of vascular disease, thrombosis, epilepsy and behavioural changes. In the forties and fifties magnesium was widely used to prevent epilepsy but now anti-epileptic drugs are used. Magnesium deficiency also causes a craving for sugar. It interferes with carbohydrate metabolism and contamination with excess flouride increases any deficiency in pill users as the flouride ion binds with magnesium.

Manganese

Nuts 3.5 to 0.7   Barley 1—8   Buckwheat 1.3
Split peas 1.3

This is likely to be lowered by pill use as vitamin B_6, folic acid, and essential fatty acids are required for manganese absorption and usage. It is essential for correct brain function and may be very low in the hair of hyperactive children and epileptics.

Iodine

Kelp 150,000   Clams 90   Prawns 65   Haddock 62

The pill can upset thyroid function as protein bound iodine and thyroxine is increased.[19] In theory, metabolic and hormone feed-back mechanisms can increase the risk of myxoedema goitre or hyperthyroidism in susceptible women.

Chromium

Yeast 112   Beef 57   Liver 55   Wheat 42

This is involved in carbohydrate metabolism, glucose
tolerance and diabetes. There has been an increase in childhood diabetes, especially in social class 1. It is possible that
this could be the result of the fact that pill taking has been
more common in higher social class mothers. Blood concentration is not a good indicator of chromium status but hair or
sweat analylis usually shows deficiencies among individuals
consuming a low protein, high sugar diet. Chromium con-
centrates ten to a hundred times in the tissues. Pregnancy
and stress decrease hair chromium levels so it is likely that
the pill induces chromium deficiency. Patients with arterio-
sclerosis are more likely to be deficient.

Selenium

Butter 146   Herring 141   Roe 123   Wheat germ 111

Low selenium levels in soil have been found in areas where
women have a high risk of breast cancer. It is possible that
selenium helps to prevent the growth of oestrogenic mycotoxins. Too high levels of selenium from supplements or
shampoos are toxic but I have seen very low levels in women
with breast disease.

Vitamins

Abnormalities in the new-born can be caused by too high or
too low levels of vitamins. There are several reasons why oral
contraceptive steroids alter vitamin metabolism. Steroids
change protein building and breakdown in the liver and
change the levels of the proteins in the blood that carries the
vitamins to the body tissues. The pill can alter the actions of
the enzymes which need vitamins to function properly.

Pill-induced nutritional upsets and allergies can threaten future pregnancies for months and even years after the pill is discontinued. The pill's interference with protein and vitamin metabolism is especially undesirable in countries where malnutrition is endemic. Lower social class or malnourished women have more risk of giving birth to an abnormal baby and they are more likely than well-fed women to develop clinical signs and symptoms of nutritional deficiencies if they are given the pill[20,21,22].

(Figures show approximate vitamin content of food in milligrams per 100 grams edible portion as published by Mineralab.)

Vitamin A

Vitamin A is stored in the liver, mostly in the form of retinol. Lamb's liver contains 50,000 International Units per 100 grams edible portion while white fish contains 2,260. Vegetable vitamin A (mostly carotene) is converted in the gut and liver, with the help of zinc, into a readily usable active form. Rich sources are red chilli peppers (21,600) and carrots (11,000). Retinol is released from the liver stores by being attached to a carrying protein, again with the help of zinc. When there is a shortage of zinc, common in pill takers, the stored Vitamin A can, in theory, build up in the liver to toxic levels.

Vitamin A levels rise during a normal menstrual cycle and towards the end of pregnancy. Lower social class women have the lowest levels, especially during the winter.

A wide range of oral contraceptives has been found to raise blood vitamin A levels, especially retinol and its transporting protein. However carotenoid levels may be lowered.

Some women still have too high vitamin A levels three months after stopping the pill and particularly high levels have been recorded in mothers who gave birth to babies with central nervous system abnormalities. The babies also had high vitamin A levels in their livers.

Vitamin A is essential for healthy eyes, hair, skin, teeth and good bone structure. It is involved in appetite, digestion, the making of red and white blood cells and in the production of sex hormones. Upsets in Vitamin A metabolism in animals can result in offspring with brain and eye defects and urogenital problems such as deformed penis and undescended testicles.

Vitamin A is essential for the integrity of mucous membranes. Pill changes in vitamin A metabolism may be one reason why thrush or candida is so common among pill users.

The B-complex vitamins

In nature if a food contains one B vitamin it usually contains the other B-complex vitamins. They interact in the body and excessive intake of one member of the group can create a deficiency of the others. Unfortunately, by far the best form of natural source is yeast, and pill users are especially likely to develop an allergy to yeast or suffer from thrush. Nowadays great care is taken to ensure that supplements of B vitamins do not contain yeast so that headaches, migraine or other reactions are not induced.

Vitamin B_1 (thiamine)

Yeast 15.6   Wheat germ 2   Sunflower seeds 2   Nuts 1

The absorption of vitamin B_1 is reduced when there is folate deficiency which can occur among pill users. The metabolism of thiamine is upset by steroids and pill users may have reduced B_1 levels in their red and white blood cells. The changes in the white cells reverse more quickly after stopping taking the pill than the changes in the red cells.

B_1 helps to convert glucose into energy or fat and to reconvert waste products from this process into useful substances.

Deficiency can cause muscle weakness, aching and stiffness, and tiredness. Neuritis, neuralgia, back pain, indigestion, flatulence and constipation can occur. There may be mental symptoms and abnormal sensitivity to noise or cold.

Deficiency in animals may cause infertility or small offspring with poor learning ability.

Vitamin B₂ (riboflavin)

Vitamin B_2 (riboflavin)

Yeast 5   Liver 3   Kidney 2.5   Wheat germ 0.68

Even very low doses of combined oral contraceptives alter red cell riboflavin levels which become low after seven months and continue to fall over three years.

Experimentally the concentration of riboflavin decreases in animals as the steroid-induced metabolic changes increase enzyme activity and cellular requirement for the vitamin which becomes used up. There may be a redistribution of the vitamin between various enzyme systems so that some enzymes use more B_2 and others less than is normal. Important cleansing antioxidant mechanisms are interfered with in women pill takers.

Alcohol intake increases any deficiency which can cause broken capillaries on cheeks and nose and wrinkled and peeling lips.

In animals B_2 deficiency has caused sterility, stillbirth, reduced liver function and limb defects. Thalidomide interfered with B_2 absorption.

Limb deformities in babies have been steadily increasing over the past 15 years and, in one study, the commonest harmful event in pregnancies which ended with babies having multiple limb deformities was the ingestion of oestrogens and/or progesterones.

B_2 deficiency was the commonest vitamin deficiency affecting 57 per cent of 30 unselected patients tested by Dr Damien Downing in his York laboratories recently. Thirty per cent were deficient of B_1 and 33 per cent were B_6 deficient. Only 23 per cent of the thirty patients had normal values for all three of these B vitamins.

Nicotinamide (also known as Niacin or B_3)

Yeast 40   Rice bran 30   Wheat bran 21   Liver 17

Nicotinamide is made in the liver with the help of B_1 and B_6. As oral contraceptives can alter both of these vitamins, nicotinamide may also be affected.

Deficiency is said to be characterised by the three 'D's — dermatitis, diarrhoea and dementia. The dermatitis is common on the cheeks and is aggravated by sunlight. A coated tongue, mouth ulcers, anorexia, dyspepsia and bowel upsets can occur. mental symptoms include depression, confusion, hostility, suspicion and irrational fears.

In animals deficiency can produce cleft palate, hare lip or limb defects.

Vitamin B_6 (pyridoxine)

Yeast 3   Sunflower seeds 1.25   Wheat germ 1.15
Tuna 1

As deficiency of this enzyme was one of the first pill abnormalities to be discovered, supplementation of women pill takers has been enthusiastic to the point of inducing overdose symptoms such as headaches, pins and needles. It is now recommended that pregnant women or those hoping to become pregnant should take no more than 50mg per day. Even low dose oestrogen combined pills can lower B_6 because of altered protein pathways. Cancer inducing byproducts are excreted in the urine. So-called menopausal 'replacement' therapy is especially likely to upset B_6 metabolism. These upsets can result in psychiatric symptoms, impaired glucose tolerance test (diabetes), urinary tract cancer and dermatitis round the mouth or genitals, also twitching, tremors and leg and foot cramps. Besides the pill, cigarettes and alcohol lower B_6.

Folic Acid

Yeast 2022   Black eye peas 440   Rice germ 430
Soya 425

People under stress and pregnant women need more folic acid than usual. It helps to form red blood cells, metabolise sugar and proteins and make antibodies. Folic acid is essential for growth, cell division and healing and the normal production of RNA and DNA which control heredity and prevent cancerous changes.

Folate deficiency can be caused by a diet low in folic acid, vitamin C, zinc or proteins. Malabsorption is likely in zinc deficient states such as those induced by alcohol, smoking and pill hormones. Coeliac disease (gluten allergy) also prevents folate absorption and many women become allergic to the grass family of foods (wheat, corn and cane sugar) when taking the pill.

Many studies have found oral contraceptives can lower folate levels but only a few women develop severe deficiency with megaloblastic anaemia. Megaloblastic changes have also been found in the cells lining the cervix uteri in some pill users and 10mg folic acid per day reversed these changes, but they returned later. It was suggested that these women were susceptible to a local depletion of folate coenzymes resulting in abnormal but not malignant DNA synthesis. We now know that the cervical cancer seems to depend on the introduction of human papilloma virus (HPV).

Over supplementation with folates can cause low B_{12} status with the risk of neurological symptoms. Folate status is altered by pregnancy and some women using oral contraceptives within six months of conception have shown especially low red cell and plasma folate levels during the first three months of pregnancy. Folate levels are lower in the winter months and at the start of a contraceptive cycle.

Deficiencies in animals can cause a wide variety of congenital abnormalities including spina bifida and other central nervous system abnormalities. The remarkable results achieved by Professor Smithells and his team in reducing neural tube defects by giving a multivitamin preparation are thought to be partly due to the extra folic acid given. Central nervous system abnormalities have been very high among the lower social classes and in certain countries — especially Scotland and Northern Ireland. In these countries fewer green vegetables are eaten than in England. Spinach, kale, brocoli and sprouts are all good sources of folic acid. The increased use of refrigerators and freezers and the greater availability of a wider range of fresh produce than ever before may have contributed to the fall in central nervous system abnormalities, but the overall total of defects continues to rise. Some NHS pregnancy multivitamin supplement contains 100mg iron and some women experience vomiting and even bleeding from the gut when they take iron and discontinue supplements. Foresight recommend that iron should be taken separately, at a different time of day, from the other mineral and vitamin supplements which include a dose of zinc twice as high as the dose of iron. A recent editorial in *Hospital Update*[23] by Dr Chanarin recommends no more than 30mg elemental iron daily and not less than 200 micrograms folate.

Vitamin B₁₂ (cyanocobalamin)

Liver 104   Clams 98   Kidneys 63   Sardines 17

This vitamin may be decreased in oral contraceptive users. It is only found in animal produce and vegans may become deficient if they do not take supplements. There is a rapidly increasing fashion of vegetarianism among the young, partly for humanitarian reasons, but, in my experience, it often begins when a girl takes the pill and becomes increasingly anorexic or allergic or merely intolerant of meat — usually beef first of all. This is followed by a dislike of fish. We are finding vegetarians are also more likely to be zinc deficient and many become quite unhealthy in their child-bearing years.

Deficiency can cause pernicious anaemia, sore mouth, tongue, pain and menstrual disturbances. Severe deficiency can degenerate the spinal cord. This is very rare and a small supplement will keep a vegan from overt deficiency.

Vitamin C (ascorbic acid)

Rosehip powder 1300   Red chillis 369   Guavas 242
Red peppers 204   Oranges 50

Plasma concentrations are lowered by oral contraceptives, smoking, aspirin and tetracyclines. The dietary requirement of vitamic C is increased by the pill. The protein ceruloplasmin which carries copper and uses up vitamin C is increased by oestrogens and oral contraceptives. Lower levels of white cell and platelet vitamin C have been found which may relate to the increased risk of thrombosis. Vitamin C helps to keep the connective tissue collagen healthy and to keep the blood vessel walls intact. It protects against infections by viruses, poisons such as pesticides, toxins like lead, dangerous drugs and allergens.

Conclusion

A fashion for ignoring the upsets in minerals and vitamins caused by the pill is being superseded by a wave of enthusiasm for mineral and vitamin supplements to help women take the pill for longer. Such an approach is theoretical nonsense because the measurable abnormalities are signs of widespread disordered metabolism and hormone takers may be resistant to supplementation or easily overloaded. Young healthy girls are being subjected to gross biological insults when they are given pill steroids and only by refusing to take such powerful and dangerous chemicals can they be truly fit for future pregnancies. However, for women who have taken the pill and have now stopped, supplements can accelerate the return to normal health and help to treat yeast allergies which may be essential before conception.

APPENDIX II
Trade Names of Steroid Sex Hormones Marketed, including Oral Contraceptives

Oral Contraceptives

Progestogens

Testosterone derivatives	Combined		Sequential		Progestogen only	
	Common trade names showing mg dose					
Norethisterone acetate	Anovlar	4				
	Gynoviar 21	3				
	Norlestrin	2.5				
	discontinued					
	Loestrin 30	1.5				
	Minovlai	1				
	Orlest 21	1				
	discontinued					
	Loestrin 20	1				
	Ortho-Novum	2				
	discontinued					
Norethisterone	OrthoNovin 1/50	1				
	Norinyl-1	1				
	Norimin	1				
	Neocon 1/35	1				
	Brevinor	0.5	Binovum	0.5		
				1		
	Ovysmen	0.5	Trinovum	0.5	Micronor	0.35
				0.75		
				0.1	Noriday	0.35

Progestogen	Preparation	Dose (mg)		
Norethynodrel	Enovid *discontinued*	10		
	Conovid *discontinued*	5		
	Conovid E *discontinued*	2.5		
Ethynodiol diacetate	Metrulen *discontinued*	2		
	Conova 30	2		
	Ovulen 50 *discontinued*	1		
	Demulen *discontinued*	0.5		
		0.5		
Lynestrenol	Lyndiol *discontinued*	5	Femulen	0.5
	Lyndiol *discontinued*	2.5		
	Minilyn	2.5		
Levonorgestrel	Eugynon 50	0.5		
	Eugynon 30	0.25		
	Ovran	0.25		
	Microgynon 30	0.15		
	Ovranette	0.15	Trinordiol	0.05
				0.075
				0.125
			Logynon	0.05
				0.075
				0.125
			Neogest	0.075
			Microval	0.03
			Norgeston	0.03
Desogestrel	Marvelon	0.15		

*Combined or sequential pills contain between 0.05mg and 0.02mg ethinyl oestradiol except Norinyl and OrthoNovin which contain 0.05mg of mestranol. Higher dose oestrogen pills were discontinued because of the thrombosis risk.

Progesterone derivatives

Megestrol acetate	Volidan *discontinued*	4
Chlormadinone		
	Sequens *discontinued*	

*Megestrol acetate and Chlormadinone were discontinued because of breast tumours in dogs.

Other Hormone Preparations

Progestogens

Testosterone derivatives	Combined with oestrogens	Alone	Sequential + oestrogen
Norethisterone acetate	Controvlar 3, Norlestrin 2.5		Trisequens 1
Norethisterone		Utovlan 5	Menophase 1, 1.5, 0.75
Norgestrel	Prempak 0.5, Prempak C 0.15	Primolut N 5	
Levonorgestrel Methyl Testosterone	Mixogen 3.6		Cyclo-Progynova 1mg 0.25, Cyclo-Progynova 2mg 0.5

Progesterone derivatives	Combined with oestrogens	Progestogen alone
Progesterone		Cyclogest (suppositories) 200, 400

Progestogens	Fixed dose		Sequential — varying doses	
Medroxy progesterone acetate	Provera	5		
	Depo Provera	50		
Cyproterone acetate	Diane	2		
Dydrogesterone	Duphaston	10		
Allyloestrenol	Gestanin	5		
Hydroxyprogesterone	Depo Proluton	250		

*Combined pills contain up to 0.05mg of ethinyl oestradiol or up to 1.25mg of conjugated oestrogens.

Oestrogens

	Fixed dose		Sequential — varying doses	
Quinestrol	Estrovis	4		
Allyloestrenol	Gestanin	5		
Piperazine oestrone sulphate	Harmogen	1.5		
Dienoestrol	Hormofemin (cream)	0.025%		
Oestriol	Ortho Dienoestrol (cream)	0.01%		
	Ovestin (cream)	0.25		
Oestriol ⎫	Hormonin	0.27		
Oestrone ⎬		1.4		
Oestradiol ⎭		0.6		
Quinestradol		0.25		
Conjugated oestrogens (equine)	Pentovis	0.25	Premarin	0.625
	Premarin (cream)	0.625		1.25
				2.5
Oestradiol valerate			Progynova	1
				2
Stilboestrol	Tampovagan	0.5		

229

Glossary

Acid and alkaline phosphatases	Zinc containing enzymes which break phosphate bonds and are concerned with secretory processes and cell division. Found in the womb and elsewhere. Their widespread actions are altered by the pill hormones.
ACTH	Adreno cortico trophic hormone secreted by the pituitary which regulates adrenal steroids.
Adenomyosis	Disease condition when the womb's glandular living tissues spread into the muscles of the womb wall.
Adrenal glands	Two small glands lying above each kidney which secrete body regulating hormones, e.g. adrenaline and cortico steroids.
Adrenaline	A hormone controlling 'fight and flight' reactions.
AIDS	Acquired immune deficiency syndrome.
Aldosterone	Adrenal cortex hormone controlling salt and water metabolism.
Allergy	Exaggerated response.
Amenorrhoea	The absence of monthly bleeding.
Amines	Building blocks which make up body proteins.
Amnesia	Loss of memory.
Anabolic	Hormones which build up protein and muscle.
Androgen	Masculinising hormone, also found in small amounts in females.
Aneurysm	Distended sac at a weak point in an artery.
Anti-thrombin III	Blood factor which prevents clotting.
Arterioles	Very small arteries.
Ascorbic acid	Vitamin C.
Benign	Simple, not malignant.
Benign intracranial hypertension	Raised fluid pressure in the spaces in the brain.
Biochemistry	The chemistry of living organisms.
Cancer	Malignant growth of gland cells which may spread to other parts of the body.
Carbohydrates	Substances made from carbon, hydrogen and oxygen such as starches, sugars and cereals.
Carcinogens	Substances which can cause cancer.

Catabolic	Stress hormones which temporarily stop cell metabolism.
Cerebral	Belonging to the brain.
Ceruloplasmin	Copper carrying blood protein, raised by the pill hormones.
Cervix	Neck of the womb.
Cholesterol	Fatty substance made in the liver, adrenals, ovaries and testes from which steroid hormones are produced.
Choriocarcinoma	Highly invasive malignant change occurring in a hydatidiform mole which can develop if any products of conception remain after a miscarriage or abortion.
Coagulation	Blood clotting.
COMT	Catechol-o-methyl transferase. A copper containing enzyme which breaks down adrenaline and is altered by the pill hormones.
Congenital	From birth.
Conjugated oestrogens	A mixture of oestrogens chemically altered to be easily excreted in the urine. See Premarin.
Corpus luteum	Yellow cyst which produces ovarian hormones at the end of the normal cycle and in early pregnancy.
Cortex	Outer part of the adrenal glands which secretes steroids.
Cortisol	Adrenal steroid hormone which alters cell metabolism.
Cortisone	A steroid medicine with a cortisol-like action.
Diaphragm	Vaginal cap used to cover the neck of womb for birth control.
Dopamine	Amine derived from protein breakdown.
Dyslexia	Learning difficulties usually involving reading, spelling, writing, arithmetic and short term memory.
Dysmenorrhoea	Pelvic cramps at period times.
Endocrine	The body's hormone secretions.
Endogenous	Belonging to the body of the individual concerned.
Endometriosis	Disease condition when the glandular womb tissue has spread elsewhere in the womb or pelvis.
Endometrium	Inner lining of the womb containing secretion-bearing glands.
Enzyme	A catalyst which speeds up chemical reactions in the body.

Erosion	Rough area on the neck of the womb.
Exogenous	Not belonging to the body of the individual concerned, e.g. hormones manufactured artificially or 'natural' hormones obtained from animal or human sources.
Fallopian tubes	Two tubes attached at each corner of the womb which stretch out towards the ovaries.
Fetus	Baby before birth.
Fibroid	Benign tumour overgrowth in the womb.
Folic acid	A vitamin essential for preventing fetal abnormalities. Reduced by the pill and stress.
FSH	Egg follicle stimulating hormone.
Glutathione peroxidase	The body's only selenium containing enzyme, which is an essential part of the body's cleansing antioxidant mechanisms. It is altered by the pill hormones.
Gynaecologist	Doctor specialising in women's illnesses.
Haemorrhage	Bleeding.
hCG	Human chorionic gonadotrophic hormone produced by the developing fetus.
Histology	Study of body tissues using a microscope.
Hormone	Body's chemical messenger.
Hypertension	High blood pressure.
Hypothalamus	Part of the base of the brain which controls the endocrine system including reproduction.
Hysterectomy	Surgical removal of the womb.
Immune	Having resistance.
Intromission	Vaginal penetration during sexual intercourse.
Kaposis sarcoma	Rare vascular skin malignancy.
Lactation	Breast feeding.
Leucocyte	White blood cell.
LH	Luteinising hormone which stimulates the corpus luteum to produce progesterone after ovulation.
Libido	Interest in having sexual intercourse.
Linoleic acid	Essential fatty acid obtained in diet from vegetable oils.
MAO	Monoamine oxidase, copper containing enzyme which breaks down amines and is altered by the pill.
Megakaryocyte	Large bone marrow cell which makes the blood platelets.
Melanoma	Highly invasive black cancer which can develop in a pigmented mole on the skin.

Menopause	Age at which menstrual bleeding stops.
Menstrual	Monthly.
Metabolism	The body's chemical reactions.
Microgram	A millionth part of a gram.
Migraine	Severe headache usually accompanied by visual disturbances or sickness.
Milligram (mg)	A thousandth part of a gram.
Narcotic	Highly addictive sedating or pain killing drugs.
Obstetrician	A doctor who specialises in pregnancy and childbirth.
Oestradiol	A natural oestrogen.
Oestrogen	Feminising hormone.
Oral contraceptive	Female hormones altered to be effectively absorbed when given as pills.
Osteoporosis	Thinning of bone structure.
Ovaries	Two hormone and egg producing glands lying in the pelvis.
Ovulation	Release of an egg from an ovary.
Pancreas	Gland lying behind the stomach which makes digestive juices.
Pathology	The study of body tissues.
Pharmacology	The study of medicines.
The 'pill'	Usually a mixture of a progestogen and an oestrogen.
Pituitary	Endocrine gland attached to the base of the brain.
Platelet	Tiny blood cells involved in clotting.
Placenta	Highly vascular structure attaching the fetus to the mother's womb.
Prednisone	A steroid medicine which acts like cortisol.
Premarin	Conjugated oestrogens obtained from the urine of pregnant mares.
Premenstrual	A few days before a period.
Progesterone	Female steroid sex hormone which prepares for pregnancy.
Progestogen	Manufactured hormone which acts like progesterone. Called 'progestin' in America.
Prostaglandin	Chemicals which help to control vascular reactions, mood and immunity.
Prostate	Male gland which secretes chemicals into semen.
Psychiatrist	Doctor specialising in mental illness.
Psychosis	Madness, loss of reality.
Pulmonary embolism	Large blood clot which has travelled from the legs or pelvic veins to the lungs.

Pyridoxine	Vitamin B_6
Renin	Kidney chemical controlling blood pressure.
Riboflavin	Vitamin B_2, part of the body's antioxidant mechanism and altered by pill hormones.
Sarcoma	Malignant growth of muscle, bone or other non-glandular tissue.
Schizophrenia	Mental illness characterised by 'split personality' with episodes of loss of reality, and often high copper and low zinc levels.
Sequential	Oral contraceptive or hormone combination when different hormones are taken on different days — usually oestrogen is taken for the first part of the month before the combined pill is started.
Serotonin	Amine derived from protein breakdown.
Sinusoid	Small veins.
Steroid	A chemical compound which has its atoms arranged in four rings and includes natural sex hormones and oral contraceptives.
Stilboestrol	Synthetic non-steroid oestrogen, known as DES (diethyl stilbestrol) in America.
Stromal condensation	A thickening of womb living tissue round the small veins.
Subarchnoid haemorrhage	Bleeding from an aneurysm in the tissues surrounding the brain.
Superficial phlebitis	Inflammation and clotting in a surface vein.
Testes	Two male glands which produce sperm and male hormones.
Testosterone	Main masculinising hormone produced in large amounts in male testes.
Thrombosis	Blood clot.
Triglycerides	Blood fats.
Tryptophan	Essential amino acid.
Uterus	Womb.
Vitamin B_6	Pyridoxine — vitamin required for the metabolism of amines. Often lowered by the pill hormones because of abnormal amine metabolism.
Zinc	Metal co-factor necessary for the correct functioning of reproduction and the immune system. Required by ninety enzymes. Lowered by the pill. Available in oysters and red meat.

References

Chapter 1
1. i) Paffenbarger, R. S. *et al* (1977) 'Cancer risk as related to use of oral contraceptives during fertile years.' *Cancer* 39, suppl. 1887
    ii) Pike, M. C. *et al* (1981) 'Oral contraceptive use and early abortion as a risk factor for breast cancer in young women.' *British Journal of Cancer* 43, 72
    iii) Harris, N.V. *et al* (1982) 'Breast cancer in relation to patterns of oral contraceptive use.' *American Journal of Epidemiology* 118, 643
    iv) McPherson, K. *et al* (1983) 'Oral contraceptives and breast cancer.' *Lancet* 2, 1414
    v) Olsson, H. *et al* (1985) 'Oral contraceptive use and breast cancer in young women in Sweden'. *Lancet* 1, 748
    vi) Rosenbergh, L. *et al* (1984) 'Breast cancer and oral contraceptive use'. *American Journal of Epidemiology* 119, 167
2. Janerich, D. T. *et al* (1977) 'Benign Breast Disease and Oral Contraceptive Use.' *JAMA* 237, 20, 2199
3. Oral contraceptives (1963) *BMJ* 2, 489 and 550
4. Seaman, B. and Seaman, G. *Women and the Crisis in Sex Hormones* Bantam Books, New York 1977

Chapter 2
Part 1
1. Mears, E. and Grant, E. C. G. (1962) 'Anovlar as an oral contraceptive.' *BMJ* 2, 75
2. Grant, E. C. G. (1965) 'Relation of arterioles in the endometrium to headaches from oral contraceptives.' *Lancet* 1, 1143
3. Grant, E.C.G. (1968) 'Relation between headaches from oral contraceptives and development of endometrial arterioles.' *BMJ* 3, 403
4. Sommervile, B. (1971) 'Daily variation in plasma levels of progesterone and estradiol throughout the menstrual cycle.' *American Journal of Obstetrics and Gynecology* 111, 3, 419
5. Grant, E. C. G. (1978) 'Creatures of the Moon.' *BMJ* 1, 165
6. Grant, E. C. G. (1964) 'The effects of oral contraceptives on the endometrium.' *Journal of Reproducion and Fertility* 8, 275
7. Grant, E. C. G. (1967) 'Hormone balance of oral contraceptives.' *Journal of Obstetrics and Gynaecology of the British Commonwealth* 74, 6, 908

8. Mears, E. *et al* (1969) 'Preliminary evaluation of four oral contraceptives containing only progestogens.' *BMJ* 2, 730

Part 2
1. Jordon, W. M. (1961) 'Pulmonary embolism.' *Lancet* 2, 1146
2. Grant, E. C. G. (1969) 'Venous effects of oral contraceptives.' *BMJ* 4, 73
3. Wright, H. P. in *Medical Physiology and Biophysics* ed. Ruch and Fulton, W. B. Saunders, Philadelphia. 1960
4. Little, K. *Bone Behaviour* Academic Press, London 1973
5. Irey, N. S., Manion, W. C., & Taylor, H. B. (1970) 'Vascular lesions in women taking oral contraceptives.' *Archives of Pathology* 89, 1
6. Osterholzer, H. O. *et al* (1977) 'The effect of oral contraceptive steroids on branches of the uterine artery.' *Obstetrics and Gynecology* 49, 2, 227
7. 'Changing oral contraceptives.' (1969) *BMJ* 4, 789
8. Inman, W. H. W. *et al* (1970) 'Thromboembolic disease and the steroidal content of oral contraceptives: a report to the Committee on Safety of Drugs.' *BMJ* 2, 203
9. Bottiger, L. E. *et al* (1980) 'Oral contraceptives and thromboembolic disease. Effect of lowering oestrogen content.' *Lancet* 1, 1097
10. Bickerstaff, E. R. *Neurological complications of oral contraceptives*, Clarendon, Oxford, 1975
11. Walsh, F. B. *et al* (1965) 'Oral contraceptives and Neuro-ophthalmologic interest.' *Archives of Ophthalmology* 74, 628
12. Wynn, V. *et al* (1982) 'Effect of duration of low-dose oral contraceptive administration on carbohydrate metabolism.' *American Journal of Obstetrics and Gynecology* 142, 6, 739

Part 3
1. Grant, E. C. G. & Mears, E. (1967) 'Mental effects of oral contraceptives.' *Lancet* 2, 945
2. Grant, E. C. G. & Pryse-Davies, J. (1968) 'Effects of oral contraceptives on depressive mood changes on endometrial monoamine oxidase and phosphatases.' *BMJ* 3, 777
3. Vessey M. P. *et al* (1976) 'A long term follow-up study of women using different methods of contraception; an interim report.' *Journal of Biosocial Science* 8, 373
4. Dalton, K. *The Premenstrual Syndrome*, Wm. Heinemann Medical Books. London 1964
5. Cohen, S. *et al* (1964) 'Histochemical studies on the human endometrium.' *Lancet* 2, 56
6. Southgate, J., Grant E. C. G. *et al* (1968) 'Cyclical variations in endometrial monoamineoxidase: Correlations of histochemical and quantitative biochemical assays.' *Biochemical Pharmacology* 17, 721

7. Michael, R. P. (1976) 'Hormones and sexual behaviour in the female.' *Hospital Practice* 10, 69
8. Holding, T. A. *et al* (1977) 'Parasuicide in Edinburgh — a seven year review 1968-74.' *British Journal of Psychiatry* 130, 534
9. Wexler, L. *et al* (1978) 'Suicide attempts 1970-75: Updating a United States Study and comparisons with international trends.' *British Journal of Psychiatry* 132, 180
10. Hawton, K. & Catalan, J. (1981) 'Psychiatric management of attempted suicide patients.' *British Journal of Hospital Medicine* 25, 4, 365
11. Ramcharan, S. *et al*. The Walnut Creek Contraceptive Drug Study. 'A prospective study of the side effects of oral contraceptives, III.' *Center for Population Research Monograph*, NIH, Bethesda 1981
12. RCGP Oral Contraception Study (1981) 'Further analysis of mortality in oral contraceptive users.' *Lancet* 541 and Kay, C. R. (1984) 'Clinics in Obst. and Gyn.' 11, 3, 759
13. McClure, G. M. G. (1984) 'Recent trends in suicide amongst the young.' *British Journal of Psychiatry* 144, 134
14. Pfeiffer, C. C. In *Mental and Elemental Nutrients*, Keats, Conn. 1975
15. Grant, E. C. G. 'Allergies, smoking and the contraceptive pill.' In *Biological Aspects of Schizophrenia and Addiction*, ed. G. Hemmings, J. Wiley, Chichester 1982

Chapter 3

1. Weindling, H. and Henry, J. B. (1974) 'Laboratory tests altered by "The Pill".' *JAMA* 229, 1762
2. 'Recent advances in oral contraception (1984).' *The British Journal of Family Planning* suppl. 10, 1, 1
3. Back, D. G. *et al* (1984) 'Pharmacokinetics and potency of contraceptive steroids.' *Lancet* 1, 171

Chapter 4

1. Volans, G. N. & Castledon, C. M. (1976) 'Relationship between smoking and migraine.' *Postgraduate Medical Journal* 52, 80
2. Grant, E. C. G. *et al* (1978) 'Oral contraceptives, smoking and ergotamine in migraine.' In *Current Concepts in Migraine Research*. ed. R. Greene, Raven Press, New York, 1978
3. Grant, E. C. G. & Clifford Rose, F. 'Smoking and Migraine.' In *Smoking and Arterial Disease* ed. R. M. Greenhalgh, Pitman Medical, London 1981
4. Petitti, D. B. & Wingerd J. (1978) 'Use of oral contraceptives, cigarette smoking and risk of subarachnoid haemorrhage.' *Lancet* 2, 234

5. RCGP (1981) 'Further analyses of mortality in oral contraceptive users.' *Lancet* 1, 541
6. Vessey, M. P. *et al* (1981) 'Mortality in oral contraceptive users.' *Lancet* 1, 549
7. Grant, E. C. G. (1983) 'Cervical cancer and oral contraceptives.' *Lancet* 1, 528
8. Hanington, E. (1967) Preliminary report on tyramine headache. *BMJ* 1, 1007
9. Grant, E. C. G. (1978) 'Oral contraceptives, smoking, migraine and food allergy.' *Lancet* 2, 581
10. Hanington, E. *et al* (1982) 'Platelet aggregation in response to 5HT in migraine patients taking oral contraceptives.' *Lancet* 1, 967

Chapter 5
1. Kalland, T. & Forsberg, J. G. (1981) 'Estrogen and Immunity.' *Journal of Immunology* 124, 2993
2. Editorial (1969) Oral contraceptives and Immune response. *JAMA* 209, 3, 410
3. Arnason, B. G. & Richman, D. P. (1969) 'Effect of oral contraceptives on experimental demyelinating disease.' *Arch. Neurol.* 21, 103
4. Grant, E. C. G. (1983) 'The contraceptive pill: Its relation to allergy and illness.' *Nutrition and Health* 2, 33
5. Grant, E. C. G. *et al* 'Hormones and headaches in women.' In *Background to Migraine* 6th Migraine Symposium Migraine Trust. London 1974
6. Mackarness, R. *Not all in the Mind* Pan, London 1976.
7. Randolph, T. G. *Human Ecology and Susceptibility to the Chemical Environment* C. C. Thomas, Illinois 1962
8. Grant, E. C. G. (1979) 'Food Allergies and Migraine.' *Lancet* 1, 966
9. Lord, G. D. A. & Duckworth, J. W. (1977) 'Immunoglobulin and complement studies in migraine.' *Headache* 17, 163
10. Fennell, P. G. S. (1983) 'Cytotoxic test for food intolerance.' *Lancet* 1, 989
11. Capel, I. D., Grant E. C. G. *et al* (1979) 'Disturbed liver function in Migraine patients.' *Headache* 19, 5, 270
12. Saunders, J. B. *et al* (1981) 'A twenty-year prospective study of cirrhosis.' *BMJ* 282, 263
13. Horrobin, D. (1984) 'Prostaglandins and essential fatty acids. A new approach to the understanding and treatment of alcoholism.' *Psychiatry in practice* 3, 21, 19
14. Abraham, G. E. (1980) 'Premenstrual tension.' *Current problems in Obstetrics and Gynecology* III, 1
15. Editorial (1969), 'Oral contraceptives and immune responses.' *JAMA* 209, 3, 410

16. Joshi, U. M. *et al* (1971) 'Effect of steroidal contraceptives on antibody formation in the human female.' *Contraception* 3, 327
17. Hagen, C. & Froland, A. (1972) 'Depressed lymphocyte response to PHA in women taking contraceptives.' *Lancet* 1, 1185
18. Beaumont, J. L. *et al* (1979) *see* Chapter 7, Ref 29
19. Miller, J. B. (1977) 'A double-blind study of food extract injection therapy: A preliminary report.' *Annals of Allergy* 38, 3, 185
20. Truss, C. O. (1982) 'The role of candida albicans in human illness.' *Journal of Orthomolecular Psychiatry* 10, 4, 228
21. Mason, P. *et al* (1984) 'Induction of ovulation with pulsatile luteinising hormone releasing hormone.' *BMJ* 288, 181

Chapter 6

1. Ramcharan, S. *et al*. The Walnut Creek Contraceptive Drug Study. 'A prospective study of the side effects of oral contraceptives, III.' *Center for Population Research Monograph*, NIH, Bethesda 1981
2. RCGP *Oral Contraceptives and Health*, Pitman Medical Books, London 1974
3. Vessey, M. P. *et al* (1976) 'A long term follow-up study of women using different methods of contraception: an interim report.' *Journal of Biosocial Science* 8, 373
4. Vaughan, Paul *The Pill on Trial*, Weidenfeld and Nicolson, London 1970
5. RCGP Oral Contraception Study (1981) 'Further analyses of mortality in oral contraceptive users.' *Lancet* 1, 541
6. Grant, E. C. G. (1974) 'Stopping the Pill.' *BMJ* 3, 115
7. Beral, V. (1974) 'Oral Contraceptives and Health.' *Lancet* 1, 1280
8. RCGP (1977) 'Mortality among oral contraceptive users.' *Lancet* 2, 727
9. Vessey, M. P. (1980) 'Female hormones and vascular disease — An epidemiological overview.' *The British Journal of Family Planning* 6, 3, 1
10. Vessey, M. P. *et al* (1981) 'Mortality in oral contraceptive users.' *Lancet* 1, 549

Chapter 7

1. Schwallie, P. C. & Mohberg, N. R. (1977) 'Medroxyacetate, an injectable contraceptive.' *Advanced Planned Parenthood* 12, 149
2. Rinaldo, C. R. *et al* (1980) 'Mechanism of immunosuppression in cytomegalovirus mononucleosis.' *Journal of Infectious Diseases* 141, 488
3. Detels, R. *et al* (1983) 'Relation between sexual practices and T-cell subsets in homosexually active men.' *Lancet* 1, 609

4. i) 'Cervical carcinoma and the pill: a possible link?' (1968) *World Medicine* 4, 6, 1

   ii) Melamed, M. R. *et al* (1969) 'Prevalence rates of uterine cervical carcinoma in situ for women using the diaphragm or oral contraceptives.' *BMJ* 3, 195

5. Grant, E. C. G. (1982) Oral Contraceptives and Malignancy. *Clinical Oncology* 8, 2, 97

6. Bamford, P. N. *et al* (1982) 'Changing pattern of cervical intraepithelial neoplasia seen in a family planning clinic.' *Lancet* 1, 747

7. Vessey, M. P. *et al* (1983) 'Neoplasia of the cervix uteri and contraception — a possible adverse effect of the pill.' *Lancet* 2, 930

8. Wright, N. H., Vessey M. P. *et al* (1978) 'Neoplasia and dysplasia of the cervix uteri and contraception: A possible protective effect of the diaphragm.' *British Journal of Cancer* 38, 273

9. Kay, R. C. (1983) 'Oral contraceptives and cancer.' *Lancet* 2, 1018

10. Robinson, J. 'Cancer of the cervix: occupational risks of husbands and wives and possible prevention strategies.' In *Pre-clinical Neoplasia of the Cervix* RCOG, London, 1982

11. British Gynaecological Cancer Group (1981) 'Oestrogen replacement and endometrial cancer.' *Lancet* 1, 1359

12. Pike, M. C. *et al* (1983) 'Breast cancer in young women and use of oral contraceptives, possible modifying effect of formulation and age of use.' *Lancet* 2, 926

13. Vessey, M. P. *et al* (1971) 'Investigation of the possible relationship between oral contraceptives and benign and malignant breast disease.' *Cancer* 28, 1395

14. Swyer, G. I. M. (1983) 'Oral contraceptives and cancer.' *Lancet* 2, 1018

15. Gillmer, M. D. G. (1983) 'Breast cancer and oral contraceptives.' *Lancet* 2, 1145

16. RCGP (1981) 'Breast cancer and oral contraceptives: findings in the Royal College of General Practitioner's Study.' *BMJ* 282, 2089

17. Vessey, M. P. *et al* (1981) 'Breast cancer and oral contraceptives: findings in Oxford/FPA Study.' *BMJ* 282, 2093

18. Stadel, B.V. *et al* (1985) 'Oral contraceptives and breast cancer in young women.' *Lancet* 2, 970

19. Tokunga, M. *et al* (1979) 'Malignant breast tumours among atomic bomb survivors, Hiroshima and Nagasaki'. *Jour. Nat. Cancer Inst.* 62, 1347

20. Greenberg, E. R. *et al* (1984) 'Breast cancer in mothers given diethylstilbestrol in pregnancy' *New England Journal of Medicine* 311, 1393

21. Report of the panel of persons appointed by the Licensing Authority to hear the application by Upjohn Ltd for a product licence to market

the drug Depo-Provera as a long-term contraceptive. Department of Health and Social Security Crown Copyright. 1984

22. 'Rejecting Scientific advice (1982)' *BMJ* 284, 1426
23. Yovich, J. L. *et al* (1983) 'Medroxyprogesterone in in-vitro fertilisation *Lancet* 1, 711
24. Grant, E. C. G. (1984) 'Cancer and the Pill.' *The Ecologist* 14, 2, 68
25. Walnut Creek Study *see* Chapter 6, Ref 1.
26. Ory, H. W. (1982) 'Non-contraceptive health benefits of pill use.' *Family Planning Perspectives* 14, 4, 182
27. The Centers for Disease Control Cancer and Steroid Hormone Study (1983). 'Oral contraceptives and endometrial cancer.' *JAMA* 249, 12, 1600
28. Cramer, D. W. *et al* (1982) 'Ovarian cancer and talc: a case-control study.' *Cancer* 50, 372
29. The Centers for Disease Control Cancer and Steroid Hormone Study (1983). 'Oral Contraceptive use and the risk of ovarian cancer.' *JAMA* 249, 17, 1596
30. Schoental, R. Carcinogens in plants and micro organisms. In *Chemical Carcinogens* ed. C. E. Searle. Am. Chem. Soc. Monogr., 173. Washington 1976, p. 626
31. Schoental, R. (1976) 'Hazards of oral contraceptives to future generations.' *International Journal of Environmental Studies* 9, 81
32. Paffenbarger, R. *see* Chapter 1, Ref 1
33. Beaumont, J. L. *et al* (1979) 'Anti-ethinyloestradiol antibody activities in oral contraceptive users.' *Clinical and Experimental Immunology* 38, 445
34. Capel, I. D. *et al* (1981) 'The effect of prolonged oral contraceptive steroid use on erythrocyte glutathione peroxidase activity.' *Journal of Steroid Biochemistry* 14, 729
35. Fasal, E. *et al* (1975) 'Oral contraceptives as related to cancer and benign lesions of the breast.' *Journal of the National Cancer Institute* 55, 4, 767
36. Jick, H. *et al* (1980) 'Oral contraceptives and breast cancer.' *American Journal of Epidemiology* 112, 5, 577
37. MacMahon, B. *et al* (1970) 'Age at first birth and breast cancer risk.' *Bulletin of the World Health Organisation* 43, 290
38. Drife, J. O. (1981) 'Breast Cancer, pregnancy and the pill.' *BMJ* 283, 778
39. Kaufman, D. W. *et al* (1984) Non-contraceptive oestrogen use and the risk of breast cancer. *JAMA* 252, 1, 63
40. Daniel, D. G. *et al* (1967) 'Puerperal thromboembolism and suppression of lactation.' *Lancet* 2, 287
41. Lingeman, C. H. (1979) 'Hormones and hormonominetic compounds in the etiology of cancer.' In *Recent Results of Cancer Research* 66, 1

241

42. Davies, J. M. (1981) 'Testicular cancer in England and Wales: some epidemiological aspects.' *Lancet* 1, 928
43. Coope, J. (1984) 'Menopause: associated problems. *BMJ* 289, 970-1
44. Finkenstedt, G. *et al* (1986) 'Lactose absorption, milk consumption and fasting blood glucose concentrations in women with idiopathic osteoporosis'. *BMJ*, 292, 161
45. Editorial (1985) 'Risk factors in postmenopausal osteoporosis'. *Lancet* 1, 1370
46. Stampfer, M. J. *et al* (1985) 'A prospective study of postmenopausal estrogen therapy and coronary heart disease'. *New England Journal of Medicine* 313, 17, 1044
47. Wilson, P. W. F. *et al* (1985) 'Postmenopausal estrogen use, cigarette smoking and cardiovascular morbidity in women over 50'. *New England Journal of Medicine* 313, 17, 1038
48. Selby, P. L., Peacock, M. (1985) 'Progestogen plus cyclical oestrogen for postmenopausal bone loss'. *Lancet* 2, 1194
49. Szmukler, G. I. *et al* (1985) 'Premature loss of bone in chronic anorexia nervosa'. *BMJ* 290, 26
50. Smith, R. *et al* (1985) 'Osteoporosis of pregnancy'. *Lancet* 1, 1178
51. Barlow, D. H. *et al* (1985) 'Effect of long-term hormone replacement on plasma prolactin concentrations in women after oophorectomy'. *BMJ* 290, 589

Chapter 8

1. Herbst, A. L. *et al* (1971) 'Adenocarcinoma of the vagina: association of maternal stilbestrol therapy with tumour appearance in young women.' *New England Journal of Medicine* 284, 878
2. Smith, O. W. (1948) 'Diethylstibestrol in the prevention and treatment of complications of pregnancy.' *American Journal of Obstetrics and Gynecology* 56, 821
3. Beral, V. & Colwell, L. (1981) 'Randomised trial of high doses of stilboestrol and ethisterone therapy in pregnancy: Long term follow-up of the children.' *Journal of Epidemiology and Community Health* 35, 155
4. Diekmann, W. J. *et al* (1953) 'Does the administration of diethyl-stibestrol during pregnancy have therapeutic value?' *American Journal of Obstetrics and Gynecology* 66, 1062
5. Shepherd, J. H. *et al* (1979) 'Cervical carcinoma in situ in a woman exposed to diethylstilboestrol "in utero".' *BMJ* 3, 246
6. Schoental, R. 'Behavioural and other effects of secondary meta-bolites of certain fusarium species.' In *Behavioural Models and the Analysis of Drug Action*. Proc. of the 27th OHOLO confer. Israel. Eds. Spiegelstein and Levy. Elsevier Scientific Pub. Co. Netherlands. 1982

7a. Matlai, P. & Beral, V. (1985) 'Trends in congenital malformations in external genitalia.' *Lancet* 1, 108.

7b. Depue, R. H., Pike, M. C. & Henderson, B. E. (1985) 'Oestrogen exposure during gestation and risk of testicular cancer'. *Jour. Nat. Cancer Inst.* 71, 6, 1151

8. Delanoe, D. *et al* (1984) 'Androgenisation of female partners of men on medroxyprogestrone acetate/percutaneous testosterone contraception.' *Lancet* 1, 276

9. Kirkwood, K. *et al* (1983) 'Oral contraceptive use and the occurrence of pituitary prolactinoma.' *JAMA* 249, 16, 2204

10. Dodds, E. C. (1961) 'Rhyme and reason in endocrinology.' *Journal of Endocrinology* 23, 3

11. Lodge Rees, E. (1981) 'The Concept of Preconceptual Care.' *International Journal of Environmental Studies* 17, 37

12.   i) Grant, E. C. G. (1981) 'The harmful effects of common social habits, especially smoking and using oral contraceptive steroids on pregnancy.' *International Journal of Environmental Studies* 17, 57

  ii) Grant, E. C. G. (1982) 'Environmental and pollutional effects upon the learning skills of young children.' *Dyslexia Review* 5, 1, 29

  iii) Grant, E. C. G. (1983) 'Recent advances in understanding toxic and teratogenic effects of hormones.' In *The Next Generation: Avoiding damage before birth in the 1980s* Foresight

13. The Association for the Promotion of Pre-conceptual care. *Guidelines for Future Parents* Foresight, Witley, Surrey. 1984

14. Capel, I. D., Grant, E. C. G. *et al* (1981) 'Comparison of concentrations of some trace, bulk and toxic metals in the hair of normal and dyslexic children.' *Clinical Chemistry* 27, 879.

15. Rimland, B. & Larson, G. E. (1983) 'Hair mineral analysis and behavior: An analysis of 51 studies.' *Journal of Learning Disabilities* 16, 5, 1.

16. Davies, S. 'Zinc nutrition and health.' In *The Yearbook of Nutritional Medicine* ed J. Bland. Keats, New Cannan, Conn. 1984

17. Barnes, B. & Colquhoun, J. *The Hyperactive Child — What the family can do*, Thorsons, Wellingborough, Northamptonshire. 1984

18. Bryce-Smith, D. 'Environmental influence on prenatal development.' In *The Next Generation: Avoiding damage before birth in the 1980s* Foresight, Witley, Surrey. 1983

19. Hurley, L. S. (1968) 'The consequences of fetal impoverishment.' *Nutrition Today* 3, 2

20. Oberleas, D. *et al* (1972) 'Trace elements and behaviour.' *International Review of Neurobiology* Suppl. 1, 83

21. Beach, R. S. *et al* (1983) 'Persistent immunological consequences of gestational zinc deprevation.' *American Journal of Clinical Nutrition* 38, 579

22. Rimland, B. & Larson, G. E. (1981) 'The manpower quality decline.' *Armed Forces and Society* 8, 1, 21

23. Goh, K. G. (1967) 'Chromosomal breakages in women taking birth control pills.' SS AFC (Report) Oak Ridge Ass. Universities, 106, 97

24. Bala Krishna Murthy, P. & Prema, K. (1979) 'Sister-chromatid exchanges in oral contraceptive users.' *Mutation Research* 68, 149

25. Lejeune, J. & Prieur, M. (1979) 'Oral contraceptives and Trisomy 21: A retrospective study of 730 cases.' *Annals of Genetics* 22, 2, 61.

26. Vessey, M. P. *et al* (1979) 'Outcome of pregnancy in women using different methods of contraception.' *British Journal of Obstetrics and Gynaecology* 86, 548

27. Gal, I. (1973) 'Variations in the incidence of congenital malformations in spontaneous abortions, stillbirths and artificially interrupted pregnancies.' *Human Genetics* 20, 367.

28. Gal, I. *et al* (1967) 'Hormonal pregnancy tests and congenital malformations.' *Nature* 216, 83

29. Nora, J. J. *et al* (1978) 'Exogenous progestogen and estrogen implicated in birth defects.' *JAMA* 240, 9, 837

30. McCredie, J. *et al* (1983) 'Congenital limb defects and the pill.' *Lancet* 2, 623

31. Robertson, W. F. (1962) 'Thalidomide (Distaval) and vitamin B deficiency.' *BMJ* 1, 792

32. Capel, I. D. *et al* (1980) *see* Chapter 7, Ref 34

33. Jofen, J. 'Long-range effects of medical experiments in concentration camps (the effect of administration of estrogen to the mother on the intelligence of the offspring).' In *The Fifth World Congress of Jewish Studies*, Jerusalem 2, 55 1972

34. Potts, M. *et al* (1982) 'The Puerto Rico oral contraceptive study: An evaluation of methodology and results of a feasibility study.' *The British Journal of Family Planning* 7, 99

35. Saenz de Rodriguez, C. A. & Toro-Sola, M. A. (1982) 'Anabolic Steroids in meat and premature telarche.' *Lancet* 1, 1300

36. Harlap, S. & Davies, M. *The Pill and Births: The Jerusalem Study* National Institute of Child Health and Development, Bethesda USA, 1978

37. Gal, I. & Parkinson, C. E. (1973) 'Changes in serum vitamin A levels during and after oral contraceptive therapy.' *Contraception* 8, 1, 13.

38. Smithels, R. W. *et al* (1980) 'Possible prevention of neural tube defects by preconceptional vitamin supplements.' *Lancet* 1, 339

39. Morley, C. J. *et al* (1982) 'Surfactant abnormalities in babies dying from sudden death syndrome.' *Lancet* 1, 1320

40. McClure, G. M. C. (1984) *see* Chapter 2, Part 3, Ref 10

41. 'Sexually transmitted disease surveillance in Britain: 1982' (1984) *BMJ*, 289, 99

42. Crook, W. G. (1983) *The Yeast Connection* Professional Books, Tennesee
43. Adler, M. W. (1983) 'Complications of common genital infections and infections in other sites, ABC of Sexually Transmitted Diseases'. *BMJ* 287, 1709
44. Singer, A. *et al* (1984) 'Genital wart virus infections: nuisance or potentially lethal?' *BMJ* 288, 735
45. Catterall, R. D. (1981) 'Biological effects of sexual freedom'. *Lancet*. 1.315
46. Hardy, P. H. *et al* (1984) 'Prevalence of six sexually transmitted disease agents among pregnant inner-city adolescents and pregnancy outcome'. *Lancet* 2, 333
47. Acheson, E. D. (1985) From the Chief Medical Officer 'The acquired immune deficiency syndrome'. *Health Trends*, 17, 75
48. Hull, M. G. R. *et al* (1985) 'Population study of causes, treatment and outcome of infertility'. *BMJ* 291, 1693
49. Davies, S. (1985) 'Effects of oral zinc supplementation on serum, hair and sweat zinc levels in seven subjects'. *The Science of the Total Environment*, 42, 45 Elsevier Science Pub. Amsterdam.
50. Campbell Brown, M. *et al* (1985) 'Zinc and copper in Asian pregnancies — is there evidence for a nutritional deficiency?' *British Journal of Obstetrics and Gynaecology* 92, 875
51. Sanstead, H. H. (1984) 'Zinc: Essentiality for Brain Development and Function'. *Nutrition Today*, 43, 5, 26
52a. Bryce-Smith, D., Simpson, R. I. D. (1984) 'Case of anorexia nervosa responding to zinc sulphate'. *Lancet* 2, 350
52b. Bryce-Smith, D. (1986) 'Environmental chemical influences on behaviour and mentation'. *Chem. Soc. Review* 15, 93
53. Adams, J. *et al* (1985) 'Multifollicular ovaries: Clinical and endocrine features and response to pulsatile gonadotropin releasing hormone'. *Lancet* 2, 1404
54. Mollay, B. G. *et al* (1985) ' "Missed pill" conception: fact or fiction?' *BMJ* 290, 1474
55. Blum, M. and Pery, J. (1985) 'The need for ovulation detection before prescribing oral contraception'. *British Journal of Sexual Medicine*, 12, 5, 126

Chapter 9
1. Vessey, M. P. *et al* (1976) 'A long-term follow-up study of women using different methods of contraception: an interim report.' *Journal of Biosocial Science* 8, 373
2. Jarrett, J. C. & Spellacy, W. N. (1983) 'Contraceptive Practices of Female Runners.' *Fertility and Sterility* 39, 374

3. Schangold, M. M. & Levine, H. S. (1983) 'The Effect of Marathon Training on Menstrual Function.' *American Journal of Obstetrics and Gynecology*, 143, 862

4. Flynn, A. & Brooks, M. *A Manual of Natural Family Planning*, George Allen and Unwin, London 1984

5. *The Billings Method*, Dr Billings, Evelyn, & Westmore, Ann, Penguin, 1982

6. World Health Organisation (1983) 'Prospective multicentre trial of ovulation method of natural family planning. Characteristics of the menstrual cycle and the fertile phase.' *Fertility and Sterility* 40, 773

7. Anon. (1983) 'Gloomy outlook for new male contraception.' *Pharmaceutical Journal* Jan. 1 and 8, 21

8. Wortman, J. S. & Sciarra, J. J. (1974) 'Control of Male Fertility: Report of a Workshop.' *Contraception* 10, 561

9. Bledin, K. D. *et al* (1984) 'Psychological sequelae of female sterilisation: short term outcome in a prospective controlled study.' *Psychological Medicine* 14, 379

10. Goldacre, *et al* (1983) 'Cardiovascular disease and vasectomy.' *New England Journal of Medicine* 308, 805

11. *Saying No Isn't Always Easy* The Responsible Society. Family and Youth Concern. Wicken, Milton Keynes 1980

12. Greer, Germaine, *Sex and Destiny*, Secker & Warburg, London 1984

Appendix I

1. Greene, R. & Dalton, K. (1953) 'The Premenstrual Syndrome.' *BMJ* 1, 1007

2. Little, K. *see* Chapter 2, Part 2, Ref 4

3. Wynn, V. & Doar, J. W. H. (1966) 'Some effects of oral contraceptives on carbohydrate metabolism.' *Lancet* 1, 715

4. Wynn, V. *et al see* Chapter 2, Part 2, Ref 12

5. i) Spellacy, W. N. *et al* (1975) 'Effects of norethindrone on carbohydrate and lipid metabolism.' *Obstetrics and Gynaecology* 45, 560

   ii) Spellacy, W. N. *et al* (1976) 'Carbohydrate and lipid metabolic studies before and after one year of treatment with ethynodiol diactate in "normal" women.' *Fertility and Sterility* 27, 900

   iii) Spellacy, W. N. *et al* (1976) 'Lipid and carbohydrate metabolic studies after one year of megestrol acetate treatment.' *Fertility and Sterility* 27, 157

   iv) Spellacy, W. N. *et al* (1981) 'Prospective studies of carbohydrate metabolism in "normal" women using norgestrel for eighteen months.' *Fertility and Sterility* 35, 167

6. Wynn, V. *et al* (1966) 'Some effects of oral contraceptives on serum-lipid and lipo protein levels.' *Lancet* 1, 720

7. Wynn, V. *et al* (1982) 'The effect of progestins in combined oral contraceptives on serum lipids with special reference to high density lipo proteins.' *American Journal of Obstetrics and Gynecology* 142, 6, 766

8. i) RCGP Oral Contraception Study (1982) 'Oral contraceptives and gall bladder disease.' *Lancet* 2, 957
    ii) Shaffer, E. A. *et al* (1984) 'The effect of a progestin on gall bladder function.' *American Journal of Obstetrics and Gynecology* 148, 504

9. Orme, M. L. E. *et al* (1984) 'Drug interactions with oral contraceptive steroids.' *British Journal of Family Planning* 10, 1, 19

10. Rose, D. P. (1966) 'Excretion of xanthurenic acid in the urine of women taking progestogen-oestrogen preparations.' *Nature* 210, 5032, 196

11. Adams, *et al* (1976) 'Influence of oral contraceptives, pyridoxine (vit. B6) and tryptohan on carbohydrate metabolism.' *Lancet* 1, 759

12. Adams *et al* (1973) 'Effect of pyridoxine hydrochloride (vit. B6) upon depression associated with oral contraception.' *Lancet* 1, 897

13. Rose, D. P & Cramp, D. G. (1970) 'Reduction of plasma tyrosine by oral contraceptives and oestrogens: a possible consequence of tyrosine amino transferase induction.' *Clinica Chemico Acta* 29, 49

14. Grant, E. C. G. *et al* 'Hormones and headaches in women.' In *Background to Migraine*, 6th Migraine Symposium, Migraine Trust, London 1974

15. Grant, E. C. G. (1975) 'The influence of hormones on headache and mood in women.' *Hemicrania* 6, 4, 2

16. Halsted, J. A. *et al* (1968) 'Plasma-zinc and copper in pregnancy and after oral contraception.' *Lancet* 2, 278

17. Fotherby, K. (1984) 'Metabolic effects of low dose combined oral contraceptives.' *British Journal of Family Planning* 10, 1, 15

18. Pfeiffer, C. C. & Iliev V. 'A study of zinc deficiency and copper excess in the schizophrenias.' In *International Review of Neurobiology* supp. 1, Academic Press, New York, 1972

19. Shatz, D. L. *et al* (1968) 'Effects of oral contraceptives and pregnancy on thyroid function.' *Canadian Medical Association Journal* 99, 882

20. *Vitamins in Human Biology and Medicine* ed Michael H. Briggs (D.Sc., Ph.D) CRC Press Inc., Florida, 1980, pp 29-64

21. Truswell Stewart, A., (1983) 'ABC of Nutrition', *BMJ* 291, 1337

22. *Supplementary chapters to Guidelines for Future Parents*, Foresight 1984

23. Chanarin, I. (1986) 'Iron Folate in Pregnancy', *Hospital Update*, March 1, 165

Useful Addresses

Action Against Allergy
Mrs Amelia Nathan Hill,
43 The Downs,
Wimbledon,
London SW20.
Tel: 01 947 5082

The Dyslexia Institute
Head Office,
133 Gresham Road,
Staines,
Middlesex TW18 2AJ.
Tel: 01 815 9498

Family Planning Information Service
Family Planning Association,
27-35 Mortimer Street,
London W1N 7RJ
Tel: 01 734 9357
*Local clinics are in the Yellow Pages of the telephone
directory.

Foresight
The Association for the Promotion of Pre-conceptual Care
Mrs Peter Barnes,
The Old Vicarage,
Church Lane,
Witley,
Godalming,
Surrey GU8 5PN.

Health Education Council
78 New Oxford Street,
London WC1A 1AH.
Tel: 01 637 1881

The Hornsby Learning Centre
71 Westside
Wandsworth Common
London SW18 2ED
Tel: 01 871 2691

Hyperactive Children's Support Group
59 Meadowside,
Angmering,
Sussex.

International Planned Parenthood Federation
18-20 Lower Regent Street,
London SW1Y 4PW.
Tel: 01 839 2911

The McCarrison Society
(nutrition and health)
76 Harley Street,
London W1N 1AE.

Natural Family Planning
NFP Centre,
Birmingham Maternity Hospital,
Queen Elizabeth Medical Centre,
Birmingham B15 2TG.
Tel: 021 472 1377 ex. 102

Index

abdomen
  bleeding of 91
  blood clots in 38
  pain in 34, 35, 54, 174
abortion 129, 139, 165—6, 199
  habitual 80, 152
  induced 177
  rates 197, 198, 199
  spontaneous 167, 168
Abraham, Prof. Guy 95
absorption
  problems 88, 93, 94, 102, 151, 182, 223
  tests 91
accidents 47, 112
  death from 58—9, 107, 110, 111
aching 221
acid phosphatase 50, 60, 215, 230
acne 66, 89
ACTH (adreno cortico trophic hormone) 206, 230
Action Against Allergy (AAA) 91, 97, 248
Adams, Dr 212—13
addiction
  alcohol 94
  allergy and 94, 96—7
  coffee 98
  drug 58, 169
  food 78
  smoking 85
adenocarcinoma of vagina 152
adenomyosis 130, 132, 230
adenosis 153, 154
adrenal glands 63, 230
  abnormal function of 145
  cancer of 142
adrenal hormones
  cortocoid 147, 230
  normal 203—14

adrenaline 156, 204, 212, 213, 230
ageing, sudden 143
age group studies 45—6, 118—19, 120, 123, 126—35, 138, 139, 150, 197
aggression 45, 47
  towards children 55—7
  towards husbands 56
AID (artificial insemination from donors) 180
AIDS (acquired immune deficiency syndrome) 117, 179—80, 199, 230
alcohol(ism) 49, 55, 58, 64, 74, 78, 79, 92, 93—7, 144, 148, 158, 164—6, 168, 169, 171, 181, 186, 194, 221—3
aldosterone 206, 217, 230
alkaline phosphatases 50, 60, 147, 150, 215, 230
alkalis 86
allergens 89—90, 93—4, 225
allergies 15, 66, 77—102, 158, 168, 216, 219, 230
  causes 79—82
  chemical 56, 64, 67, 77—8, 85—90, 93, 102, 174, 178, 211
  in children 172
  food 50, 56, 60, 64, 67, 74—5, 77—9, 84—93, 99, 102, 113, 145, 148, 151, 161, 172, 174, 178, 181, 182, 211, 220, 223, 224, 225
  and migraine 82—4, 86, 87
allyloestrenol 229
aluminium 144, 158, 159, 162
amenorrhoea 23, 29, 33, 113, 208, 230

American Journal of Obstetrics and Gynecology 153
American Society of Clinical Ecologists 85
amine(s)
  balance 156
  brain 213
  metabolism 33, 49, 51, 52, 94, 212, 230
amino acids 92, 205
amnesia 47, 96, 230
ampicillin 211
amputations 113
anabolic steroids 204, 207, 209, 210, 212, 230
anaemia 188
  copper-deficiency 164
  iron-deficiency 107, 130, 133—4, 164, 216
  megaloblastic 223
  pernicious 225
  test 25
anaesthetics 166
androgen(s) 65, 66, 142, 195, 204, 207, 209, 210, 212, 230
aneurysm 39, 230
angiotensin 206
animal(s)
  cancer in 142
  caponisation 141—2
  tests 27, 37, 52, 63, 98, 136—7, 154—6, 162—3, 172, 183, 195, 206, 221, 228
ankles, swollen 35, 55
anorexia nervosa 62—3, 65, 67, 92, 148, 160, 183—4, 216, 222, 224
Anovlar 34, 226
antenatal viral infection 178
antibiotics 23, 82, 88, 100, 174, 177, 211
antibodies 67, 80, 81, 83, 90—2, 97—8, 102, 137, 155, 179, 196—7, 223

anti-depressants 53, 73, 96, 211
anti-epileptic drugs 217
antifibrinolytic agents 188
antifungal antibiotics 100, 102
antigens 80
anti-oestrogen 207
  therapy 148
anti-oxidants 137, 172, 211, 221
antiprostaglandin agents 188
antipyrine clearance test 92—3, 215
anti-social behaviour 57
anti-thrombin III 36, 230
antizona antibodies 197
anxiety 26, 53, 54, 55, 88, 92, 99, 106
appendicitis 176
appetite 220
  loss of 62—3, 184
  see also anorexia nervosa
arterial disease 64, 210
arterial thrombosis 38, 42, 43
arterioles 28—9, 31, 134, 230
artery(ies)
  changes 32, 33, 38—9, 44, 55
  clots 34, 42
  thickened 33, 38—9
arthritis 83, 87, 88, 148, 205
  rheumatoid 104, 133
artificial insemination from donors
  see AID
aryl hydrocarbon hydroxylase (AHH) 92
ascorbic acid *see* vitamin C
aspirin 225
asthma 81, 82, 205
atherosclerosis 145, 196, 210, 218
athletes, women 189
Atkinson Morley neurosurgical hospital 43
Atlanta Centers for Disease Control 127, 132, 134, 135
atrophy 108, 114, 134, 149
Auschwitz 168—9
auto-immune disease 97, 144, 148

babies
  cot death 172, 185
  death from herpes 178
  low birth-weight 179, 182
  new-born, abnormalities in 128,
    155, 165—8, 170, 177—8,
    200, 216, 218, 219, 221
  premature 162
  STD and 177—8
  test-tube 155
  violence to 55
back
  pain 148, 221
  problems 63
bacterial flora 100, 211
bacterial infections 117, 178
Bagshawe, Professor 129
Baltimore study of pregnant
    adolescents 179
Ban the Jab 128
Barnes, Mrs Belinda 157—8, 160,
    162
barrier methods of contraception
    188, 189—90, 196, 199—
    200, 201
battered children 45, 48
Beaumont, Dr J.L. 98, 137
beef 88, 89, 224
beer 136
behavioural problems 154, 160,
    163, 168, 185, 217
benign intracranial hypertension
    42, 43, 230
Beral, Dr Valerie 109
Berer, Marge 127
Billings ovulation method of birth
    control 191—3
Binovum 226
Biolab 182, 184
biopsies 89
Birmingham Maternity Hospital
    191
birth see childbirth
birth control see contraception
birth defects 162, 184—5, 218—19,
    221

birth marks 170
bisexual reproduction 204
bladder, cancer of 142, 212
bleeding
  breakthrough 26, 33, 55, 65, 208
  from gut 224
  heavy 38, 54, 56
  irregular 32, 33, 38, 51, 54—6,
    78, 125, 129, 146, 188, 211,
    216
  miscarriage 153
  prevention of 125
  withdrawal 32, 33, 116, 134,
    141, 216
    lack of see amenorrhoea
  from womb lining 108, 114
blindness
  from birth 178
  sudden 38
blood
  cell formation 220, 223
    abnormal 44, 63, 67, 75,
      82—3, 167, 214, 220, 223
  changes 36—7, 44
  clots 33—44, 75, 80
  copper, raised levels 53, 100,
    214—15, 231
  fats 64, 65, 209, 210
  flow changes 37—8
  pressure, high 39—40, 42, 43, 55,
    86, 87, 106, 205, 206, 208,
    215
  pyruvate 209
  sugar
    low 206, 209
    raised levels 63, 205, 207
  tests 91
    AIDS virus 179
  transfusions 83, 117
  vessel
    abnormalities 117, 212, 216
    growth 204, 206, 225
    wall changes 38—40, 44, 63,
      67, 80, 209
zinc, low 100

252

body chemistry 64—5, 203—25
Bone Behaviour 205—6
bone(s)
  abnormalities in 63, 67
  formation 151
  marrow
    cells 75, 216
    transplants 91
  metabolism 144—5, 148, 205
  structure 220
  thinning of *see* osteoporosis
bowel upsets 222
boys
  born with abnormal testicles 155, 184
  precocious sexual development in 170, 185
brain
  abnormalities 167, 212, 220
  amines 213
  changes 43, 45—60, 67, 106, 173
    and womb changes 50—2
  clots 112
  damage 178
  function
    and GLA 171—2
    and manganese 217
    and zinc 160—1, 183
  haemorrhage 39, 42, 49, 200
  hormones 20—1, 63, 101, 198, 203, 206
  problems 43
  thrombosis 43
bread 84, 86
breast(s)
  cancer 13—16, 19, 111, 115—16, 122—9, 136—41, 144, 147—50, 169, 218
  development 170
  disease, hyperplastic 38, 108, 218
  enlargement 195
  feeding 178
  lumps *see* mastitis
  tenderness 26

tumours 228
Brevinor 226
British Journal of Family Planning 109
British Journal of Obstetrics and Gynaecology 181
British Medical Journal 18, 26, 52, 61, 108, 128, 143
British Society for Clinical Ecology 85—6, 98
Bryan cytotoxic test 91
Bryce-Smith, Professor Derek 162, 183
bulimia 65
Burch, Prof. Philip 134
Burn, Mr Ian 89

cadmium 120, 144—5, 158, 159, 160, 162, 167
caesarian section 179
caffeine 64
calcium 95, 144, 145, 151, 162
cancer 34, 37, 64, 67—9, 83, 103, 114, 115—51, 169, 216, 222, 223, 230
  adrenals 142
  bladder 142, 212
  breast 13—16, 19, 111, 115—16, 122—9, 136—41, 144, 147—50, 169, 218
  cervical 72—3, 76, 111, 115—16, 118—22, 128—33, 142—3, 149, 152, 177, 223
  in children 128, 152—6
  death from 110, 113, 132, 137, 150, 153
  endometrium 39, 53, 103, 111, 122, 129—34, 142, 144, 147, 149, 150
  Gentle Method of treatment 89
  kidneys 142
  liver 111, 142
  lung 111, 133, 135
  lymphoid tissue 142
  ovarian 129—33, 142, 149, 150

pituitary 142
sex hormone dependent 129—32
testicular 117, 135, 142, 155, 156, 184
thyroid 111
urinary tract 222
uterine 142
vaginal 142, 152, 184
womb 116, 147
candida albicans 100, 151, 174, 179, 181, 182, 220
candidiasis (aka thrush; monilia) 100, 173—5, 179, 220
cane sugar 89, 223
Capel, Dr Ifor 92, 137, 159, 167
caps, cervical 25, 68, 120, 135, 190, 199
carbohydrates 61, 174, 182, 210
low- diet 100
metabolism of 63—4, 67, 92, 203, 207, 209, 213, 217, 218, 230
carbon monoxide 70
carboxy haemoglobin (COHb) 70
carcinogens 92, 137, 205, 212, 230
carcinoma in situ (early cervical cancer) 118—20, 129, 152—4, 188
Cardiothoracic Institute, Brompton Hospital 90
cardiovascular disease 109, 146, 167
carotene 219
Carrol, Dr Desmond 69
Castledon, C.M. 70
catabolic steroids 205, 231
catechol oestrogens 52
cell
growth 204, 206, 216
metabolism 64, 205
central nervous system malformation 166, 171—2, 219, 223—4
cerebral artery thrombosis 42
cerebral palsy 178
cerebrovascular disease 146

ceruloplasmin 167, 214—15, 225, 231
cervicitis 175
cervix 190—2, 196, 201, 223, 231
adenosis 154
cancer 72—3, 76, 111, 115, 116, 118—22, 128—33, 142—3, 149, 152, 177, 223
caps 25, 68, 120, 135, 190, 199
carcinoma 154
chronic inflammation of 38
erosions 106, 175
infection 179, 188
mucus 32, 191—3
secretions 190
smear tests 13, 25, 118—21
Challenger, Mrs Judith 112—13
Charing Cross Hospital 83, 90, 92, 94, 129, 158, 184
Breast Clinic 89
Neurology Department 69
Special Metabolic Ward 93
cheese 49, 74, 157, 212
Chelsea Hospital for Women 195
chemical(s)
allergies 56, 64, 67, 85, 86—90, 174, 178, 211
spermicides 188—90, 199
toxic 102, 142, 164
Chemical Victims 85
chest
pain 54, 96, 148
tightness in 55
childbirth 140—1
depression after 55, 57; see also post-partum depression
exposure to hormones in 154, 173, 205
multiple 101
osteoporosis and 148
risks to mother after 37
simulation of state 56
children
anti-social behaviour in 57, 181
cancers in 128, 152—6

congenital abnormalities in 15, 135, 158—9, 162, 165—72, 177—9, 181—5, 200, 216, 218—19, 221, 223, 231
dyslexia in 159—61, 169, 181
hair mineral analysis of 160—3
homosexuality in 156—7
intelligence defects in 163—5, 168—9, 216
learning difficulties in 160—1, 163, 168—9, 172, 183, 185, 216, 221
nutrition and 157—63
precocious sexual development in 170
sick 172—3
zinc deficiency in 160—5
China, family planning in 200
chlamydia trachomatis 174—9
chlormadinone 32, 54, 115, 228
chocolate 49, 74, 88, 89, 157, 212
cholesterol 17, 18, 62, 64, 146, 169, 203, 209, 210, 231
choriocarcinomas (malignant moles) 128—9, 231
chorionic gonadotrophine (hCG) 101
chromium 65, 158, 161, 218
chromosome abnormalities 165—8, 216
cigarette smoke 86, 88
   see also smoking
circulatory deaths 110, 111, 115, 116
Clarke, Kenneth 127
cleft palate 167
clinical ecology 85—6, 97, 137, 161, 170, 195, 201
Clinical Ecology Society 137
clotting 33—44, 75, 80
   see also thrombosis
coagulation 231
coeliac disease 93, 223
coffee 78, 79, 88—90, 93, 98, 211
coil see intra-uterine device

coitus interruptus (aka withdrawal or Roman method) 199, 200
colds 175
colic, infantile 161, 178
colitis 89
   ulcerative 106
collagen 225
Colquhoun, Irene 162
combined pills 29, 31—3, 41, 44, 51, 98, 104, 116, 129, 214—26, 227—9
Committee on Safety of Drugs (CSD) 40—1, 62
Committee on Safety of Medicines 40, 124, 211
COMT (catechol-o-methyl transferase) 64—5, 213—14, 231
conception, prevention of see contraception
condoms 189
confidentiality of GPs 198
confusion 222
congenital abnormality 15, 135, 158—9, 162, 165—72, 177—9, 181—5, 200, 216, 218—19, 221, 223, 231
conjugated oestrogens 139—40, 229, 231
conjunctivitis 178, 179
Conova 227
Conovid 227
constipation 89, 221
Contracep 190
contraception
   advice to young on 197—200
   barrier methods 188—90, 196, 199—201
   caps see cervical caps
   diaphragms 45, 73, 110, 135, 175—6, 187—90, 199, 231
   IUDs see intra-uterine device
   mechanical methods 14, 25, 45, 55, 56, 68, 73, 110, 120, 135, 175, 187, 199
   for men 194—5
   natural 190—4

oral *see* pill, the
sterilization 195—7
contraceptive pill *see* pill, the
control over life, given by pill 199
Controvlar 228
convenience of pill 46, 68, 202
copper 59, 60, 64, 65, 95, 100, 146, 148, 151, 159, 160, 162, 164—5, 167, 182, 184, 214—15, 225
   intra-uterine device 56, 180, 187, 215
copulins 52
corn 89, 90
coronary artery disease 106, 146, 147
corpus luterum 231
cortex 231
corticosteroids 145, 146, 150, 205, 230
cortisol 75, 172, 205, 206, 209, 210, 212, 231
cortisone 38, 43, 85, 137, 205, 237
cot death 172, 185
Council for the Investigation of Fertility Control 14, 31, 40
cow's milk 172
Cox, Dr Hugh 201—2
cramps
  leg 37, 38, 40, 44, 54, 55, 88, 116, 222
  during pregnancy 26
creams, contraceptive 25
crime 47, 58
  violent, and low SAT scores 164
Crohn's disease 106
cultural comparisons 182
cyanide 167
cyanocobalamin *see* vitamin B_{12}
Cyclogest 228
Cyclo-Progynova 228
cyproterone acetate 229
cystic glands 115
cystitis 87—9, 190
cytomegalovirus 178

Dalton, Dr Katharina 47, 203
danazol 209
Davies, Dr Stephen 161
deafness 178
death
  from AIDS 179
  from cancer 110, 113, 120, 132, 137, 150, 153
  circulatory 110, 111
  coronary 147
  cot 172, 185
  from heart disease 70, 76
  neonatal 162
  rates of pill-users 110, 116, 120
  through suicide or accident 47, 53, 58—9, 106, 107, 110, 111
  from violence 58—9, 106, 107, 110, 111
dementia 222
Demulen 34, 227
Depo Proluton 229
Depo-Provera (DMPA) 116, 229
  Inquiry 127—8
depression 26—8, 32, 42, 45—6, 54—6, 59—61, 81, 89, 95—6, 99, 101, 107—8, 160, 164, 196, 205, 208, 212—13, 216, 222
  and MAO inhibitors 49—50
  oestrogen for 53
  post-partum 55, 57, 59, 80, 215
dermatitis 222
desensitisation 96, 99—100
desogestrel 65, 227
diabetes 134, 207—9, 216, 218, 222
Diane 229
diaphragm 45, 73, 110, 135, 175—6, 187—90, 199, 231
diarrhoea 160, 222
dienoestrol 229
diet
  bad habits 142
  high fibre 161
  and infertility 101, 180—1
  low allergy 86—90, 149, 161

low animal fat 169
and migraine 74—5, 78, 83
and PMS 30
rotation 86—90, 96, 99
diethyl stilboestrol (DES) 115, 140—3, 152—4, 156, 157, 170
digestion 220
dilated sinusoids 35—8, 54
'dipstick' birth control method 191
distended veins 32, 35—7, 44
divorce 57
dizziness 28, 54, 56, 88, 96
DMPA *see* Depo-Provera
DNA 216, 223
doctors 16, 56, 68, 97, 104, 112, 137, 141, 143, 186, 191, 192, 198, 200, 202
Dodds, Prof. Sir Charles 136, 140, 157
Doll, Prof. Sir Richard 123
dopamine 212, 213, 231
dose levels 29—35, 51, 55, 56, 125, 167, 184, 188, 211
Downing, Sir Damien 221
Down's Syndrome 165
Drife, James Owen 138—9
drowsiness 88
drug(s) 64, 96, 158, 164, 166, 225
  abuse 179
  addiction 58, 169
Dundee Medical School 16
Duphaston 229
Dydrogesterone 229
dyslexia 154, 159—61, 169, 171, 181, 183, 231
Dyslexia Institute 159, 248
dysmenorrhoea 231
dyspareunia (painful intercourse) 174, 175
dyspepsia 222
dysplasia 188

Eat Fat and Grow Thin 85

ectopic pregnancy 128, 133, 156, 175—7, 187
eczema 161
egg(s)
  as food 89—91, 136
  in ovulation 192
electrocardiogram abnormal 208
electromagnetic contraception research 201—2
Ellis, Aeronwy 91
emotional upsets 194, 205
endocrine system 164, 203, 231
endometrial sinusoids, dilated 35—7, 54
endometriosis 176, 190, 231
endometrium 31—2, 50, 147, 187, 213, 231
  cancer of 39, 53, 103, 111, 122, 129—34, 142, 144, 147, 149, 150
Enovid 19, 227
environmental units 102
enzyme(s) 34, 46, 49, 50, 64—6, 92, 142, 167, 187, 210, 214—15, 217—18, 221, 230—1
  linked isoabsorbent assay (ELISA) 90—1
  secretory 60
epilepsy 106, 211, 217
equine 229
ergotamine 71—2, 83, 86, 88, 214
erosion 232
erythromycin 178
essential fatty acids 171—2, 217
Estrovis 229
ethinyl oestradiol 40, 65, 98, 124—6, 208, 210—11, 214, 227, 229
ethynodiol diacetate 34, 54, 124, 209, 227
Eugynon 34, 227
euphoria, manic 95
evening primrose oil 95, 171
exercise 78, 144, 198
expulsion 188

eyes 43, 88, 148, 178, 220
  see also blindness, sudden

facial malformations 167
fainting 55
Falliers 98
fallopian tubes 232
  blocked 180, 188, 198
  loss of 177
families, split 55, 187
family planning
  clinics 194
  natural 190—4
  size 199, 200
  see also contraception
Family Planning Association
    22—5, 41, 45, 68, 72, 105,
    248
Fasal, Dr Elfriede 137, 138
fat metabolism 61—3, 67, 92, 94,
    171, 203, 205, 207, 209,
    210, 220
fatty acids 92, 95
feminisation of male fetuses 156,
    184
Femulen 227
fertile phases 191—4, 201
fertilisation, in-vitro (IVF) 180—1
fertility 101, 143, 180—4, 191, 194,
    195, 201, 202
fetal abnormalities 171, 172,
    199—200
fever 206
fibroids 89, 132, 148, 216, 232
fibroma 130
financial cost of pill 200—1
fingers, swollen 55
Finn, Dr Ronald 98
Fisher, Mrs Wendy 159
flatulence 221
fluoride 217
flushing 143, 148
Flynn, Dr Anna 191, 192
folate coenzyme depletion 223
folic acid 64, 120, 172, 217, 223—4,
    232

follicle stimulating hormone (FSH)
    20, 232
food
  addiction 78
  allergies 50, 56, 60, 64, 67, 77—9,
    84—93, 99, 151, 161, 172,
    174, 178, 181, 211, 223—5
  and liver function 92—3, 178
antibodies 90—2
and migraine 74—5, 84—6
Food Factor in Disease 84
Foresight, the Association for Pre-
    Conceptual Care 101,
    157—9, 162, 165, 167,
    180—1, 183, 224, 248
Framingham Heart Study Group
    146—7
Franklin, Benjamin 137
Froland, A. 197
Fulham Hospital 94
fulminating demyelining problem
    43
fungal infections 117
fungicides 136

Gal, Dr Isobel 166, 171
gall
  bladder 203
    disease 61—2, 106, 210
    stones 210
gamma-globulin 171
gamma-linolenic acid (GLA) 95,
    171
gas, domestic 86—8, 96, 99
gastro-intestinal infections 82
gender
  differences and DES 156
  and smoking 69
general practitioners (GPs) 16, 56,
    68, 97, 104, 112, 191, 197,
    198
genital
  herpes 100, 120, 173, 177—8
  itching 175
  tract malformation 156

ulceration 177—8
warts 120, 173, 177
Gestanin 229
Gillie, Oliver 176
Glen, Drs Iain and Evelyn 95
glucocorticoids 205—6, 209
glucose 205, 207, 220
  tolerance 209, 213, 218
    tests 91, 93, 145, 208, 222
glutathione peroxidase 137, 167, 172, 232
gluten, allergy to (coeliac disease) 93, 223
gonorrhoea 100, 173—6, 179, 189
grains 84, 94, 136
Greenblatt and Mishell 126
Greene, Dr Raymond 68, 203
Greer, Germaine 198—200
Grenville College 159
growth 63, 223
  hormones 67, 203, 204
Guidelines for Future Parents 158
Guillebaud, Dr John 189
gut
  bacteria 211
  bleeding 224
Guy's Hospital 42
Gynovlar 34, 226

haemophiliacs 117
haemorrhage 232
  brain 39, 49
  subarachnoid 39, 109
haemorrhagic stroke 109
haemorrhoids 35
Hagen, C. 97
hair
  abnormal growth 46, 66, 155
  healthy 220
  loss 216
  mineral analysis 158—62, 181, 187, 215, 217, 218
Halsted, J.A. (with Hackly and Smith) 214
hands, swollen 99

hangovers 95
Hanington, Dr Edda 74, 75, 84
Hare, Dr Francis 84
hare lip 167
Harmogen 229
Harvard University 19, 146, 147, 152
hay fever 81, 82, 106
hCG (hormone) 197, 232
headache 26—9, 33, 35, 39, 41—3, 49—50, 54—5, 61, 68—70, 73, 74, 77—81, 83—4, 86—8, 96, 98—9, 106—7, 208, 220, 222
  and hormonal balance 29—32
  see also migraine
heart
  abnormalities 167
  attacks 34, 70, 93, 108, 145, 196, 210, 215
  disease 64, 144, 146, 171, 196
  rate, increased 88
heat treatment for cervical erosions 118
hemoglobin 216
Henry, J.B. 65
hepatitis 92, 178
Herbst, Dr Arthur 152
hereditary defects 82, 83
herpes 100, 120, 173, 177—8
high density lipoprotein (HDL$_2$) 210
Hill, Amelia Nathan 91
Hiroshima 127
histamine 49
histology 232
homeostatic mechanisms 142
homosexuality 117, 156—7, 179
honey caps 190
Hormofemin 229
hormone(s)
  balance 22—33, 62, 99, 217
  exposure to, in utero 153—5
  and headaches 29—32
  how they work 19—21

and immune systems 78—9, 83
long-term effects on ovaries 168—9
normal adrenal 203—14
pregnancy and 20—1, 57, 79, 80, 152—7, 164—73, 184—5, 187, 205
replacement therapy (HRT) 62, 132, 143—6, 153, 187
steroid *see* pill, the
Hormonin 229
Horrobin, Dr David 95
hospital admissions 48, 55, 134, 174—5
emergency 76
referrals 188
Hospital Update 224
hostility 222
Howard, Dr John 160—1, 181, 182
human papilloma virus (HPV) 177, 223
Human Susceptibility to the Chemical Environment 86—7
Hurley, Prof. Lucille 162
hydatidiform moles 128—9
hydrocortisone 209
hydroxyprogesterone 229
Hyperactive Children's Support Group 162, 249
Hyperactive Child—What the Family Can Do, The 162
hyperactivity 154, 160, 171, 172, 181, 216, 217
hyperplastic
breast disease 38
glands 115
hypertension 39, 42, 89, 134, 196, 232
hyperthyroidism 217
hypothalamus 63, 206, 232
hysterectomy 39, 42, 44, 53, 130, 132, 134, 136, 140, 143, 147, 148, 150, 232

Iliev, V. 215

imipramine 211
immune 232
abnormalities 64, 67, 72, 83—4, 86, 216
changes 97—9, 102, 117, 137, 173, 205
systems 78—82, 89, 90, 105
immuno-deficiency 163
immunoglobin A (IgA) 82, 83, 88, 90
immunoglobin E (IgE) 81—3, 90
immunoglobin G (IgG) 82, 83, 88, 90
immunoglobin M (IgM) 82, 83, 90
immunology 197, 201
implants, hormone 196
indigestion 221
infant feeding 157—9
infantile colic 161, 178
infections 64, 80, 82, 96, 102, 106, 128, 156, 166, 172—6, 188, 205, 211, 216, 225
infertile phases 192—4
infertility 101, 113, 134, 135, 155, 156, 168, 174, 180—3, 187, 199, 221
influenza 175
injury 205, 206
Institute of Psychiatry 52
insulin
resistance to 63
secretion 205, 208—9
intelligence
declining 163—5
defects 168—9
International Migrain4 Symposium, 1978 87—90
International Planned Parenthood Federation 22, 249
intestinal villi, atrophying of 93
intra-uterine devices (IUDs) 68, 73, 120, 156, 175—7, 181, 187—8, 196
copper 56, 165
intromission 199, 232

in-vitro fertilisation (IVF) 180—1
iodine 65, 217
iron 65, 161, 214, 216
    deficiency anaemia 107, 130,
        133—4, 164, 216, 224
    supplements 172
irrational behaviour 56, 222
irritability 32, 42, 45—7, 51, 55, 205
Israeli study of teenagers 184
itching, genital 175
IUDs *see* intra-uterine devices

Jackson, Dr Margaret 194
Janerich, Prof. 166
Japanese Welfare Ministry 169
Jeffcoate, Prof. S.L. 195
Jerusalem study 128, 170
Jick, Dr Hershel 137, 138
Jofen, Prof. Jean 168—9
joints, problems with 63
Joshi, U.M. 97
*Journal of the American Medical
    Association (JAMA)* 97,
    139

Kaposi's sarcoma 117, 232
kidney(s)
    cancer of 142
    damage 40
    function 203—4, 206, 230
    transplants 91

labour 263
    induction of 154
    premature 156
lactation 128, 140—1, 148, 154,
    161, 163, 203, 216, 232
Lancet 34, 49, 75, 87, 88, 98, 109,
    119, 122, 124—7, 134, 145,
    155, 170
lead 55, 144—5, 158, 160, 162, 167,
    225
learning difficulties 160—1, 163,
    168—9, 172, 183, 185, 216,
    221

leg(s)
    blood clots in 38
    cramps 37, 38, 44, 54, 55, 88,
        116, 222
    sore 28, 35, 40, 62
Lejeune, Prof. 165
leucocyte 232
leukorrhoea 175
levonogestrel 208, 227, 228
libido 232
    increase in 35, 46, 196
    loss of 26—8, 32, 45, 46, 194—5,
        208
lice 173
limb reduction defects 166, 221,
    222
linoleic acid (LA) 95, 171, 232
Little, Dr Kitty 28, 37, 63, 75, 117,
    147, 205—6
Little of What You Fancy, A 85
liver
    cancer 11, 142
    clots 38
    damage 92, 94, 137, 168, 171,
        178
    disease 83
    function 203, 205, 207, 211, 215,
        219, 221
        and food allergies 92—3, 102,
            151
    problems 64, 65, 67, 88, 92—3,
        184, 218
    tests 91
l-norgestrel 65
Lodge Rees, Dr Elizabeth 157—8,
    160, 215
Loestrin 226
Logynon 227
London Trials, the 14, 22—61, 125
Lo/Ovral 125
Lord, Dr George 83—4, 90
lung
    cancer 111, 133, 135
    clots 34, 38

luteinising hormone (LH) 20, 101, 232
lymphocytes 98
lymphoid tissue, cancer of 142
Lyndiol 227
Lynestrenol 227

Mackarnass, Dr Richard 85—6
MacMahon, B. 138
McPherson, Dr Klim 126
magnesium 64, 65, 158, 161, 181, 217
'male pill, the' 19
malignant moles see choriocarcinomas
malnutrition 219
manganese 65, 158, 217
Mansfield, Dr 86, 91
MAO see monoamine oxidase
Margaret Pyke Centre 119, 189
Marie Curie Memorial Laboratories 92, 137
marriage break-up 57—8, 96
Marvelon 65, 227
masculinisation of female fetuses 156, 184
masking 77—9
Massachusetts General Hospital, Boston 152
mastitis 15—16, 89, 99, 111, 115, 116, 123, 171, 209
maximum mucus grading (MMG) 192
Mears, Dr Eleanor 18, 23—4, 27, 126
Medical Research Council 171, 183
medroxy progesterone 39
    acetate (MPA) 44, 229
megakarocytes 37, 232
megaloblastic anaemia 223
megestrol acetate 32, 115, 209, 228
Melamed, Dr 32, 118
melanin 132
melanoma, malignant 111, 131, 132, 232

men, contraception for 194—6
meningitis 35
menopausal depression 53
menopause 62, 140, 143, 145—7, 204—5, 233
    problems with 78, 104, 122, 129, 142, 146, 210
Menophase 228
menorrhagia 43, 134
menstrual 233
    cycle 20, 21, 29, 113, 219
    migraine 81
    problems 66, 78, 107, 144, 174, 225
menstruation 125, 184, 192, 194
    disruption of 168—9
    postponement test 124
    precocious 170
mental handicap 154
mental illness 15, 45—60, 95, 106—7, 173—4, 221—2
mental retardation 127—8, 178
mercury 144, 148, 158, 162
mestranol 32, 35, 40, 43, 54, 124, 207, 227
metabolic upsets 53, 61—7, 94, 146, 167, 169, 172, 198, 207, 212—13, 220, 222, 225
metabolism 204, 211, 218, 221, 223, 233
    progressive deterioration of 208—9
metals, toxic 100, 120, 144m, 148, 151, 158, 160—2, 167, 181
methyl testosterone 228
Metrulen 227
Michael, Dr Richard 52
microcephaly 178
microdose pills 44, 72, 126, 208, 209
Microgynon 227
Micronor 226
microthrombi (small clots) 147, 150, 205
Microval 227

Middlesex Hospital 74
migraine 14, 26—32, 36, 49, 56, 59,
        68—77, 81—4, 86—8, 90—3,
        97, 106—7, 116, 212—15,
        220, 233
Migraine Trust 68
  1974 Symposium 83
milk 87—91, 136, 145, 151
  cow's 172
  human 171
mineral(s)
  analysis 158—64, 180—4
  corticoids 206—7
  metabolism 214—18
  supplements 89, 95—6, 101—2,
        148, 158, 162, 183, 185,
        224—5
  trace 63, 65, 67, 120, 167—8,
        172, 181
Minilyn 227
Minovlai 226
miscarriage 129, 142, 152, 153,
        156, 170, 181, 183, 187
Mixogen 228
monilia (candidiasis, aka thrush)
        100, 173—5
monoamine oxidase (MAO) 46,
        48—52
  inhibitors 48—9, 60, 64, 213,
        214, 232
mood changes 27, 29, 41, 45—57,
        62, 78, 88, 108, 191, 211
mouth
  bad taste in 56
  sore 225
  ulcers 222
MPA (progesterone derivative)
        115—16, 155, 210
mucous membranes 220
Müller, Dr Bruce 83
multiple infections 179
multiple partners 176
multiple sclerosis (MS) 43—4, 80,
        97

multivitamin B preparations 101,
        224
murder committed by pill users 59
muscle
  growth 204, 230
  weakness 221
mushrooms 86, 88, 89
mutagens 137
mycoplasma hominus 179
mycotoxins 84, 102, 136, 218
myeloma 83
myocardial infection 109
myxoedema goitre 217

Nagasaki 27
nails, white spots on 216
narcotic 233
nasal catarrh 106
National Association of National
        Family Planning Teachers
        (NANFPT) 191
National Health Service (NHS) 75,
        97, 181, 201
natural family planning 190—4,
        196, 200, 249
'natural oestrogens' 39
nausea 23, 27, 56, 96, 206, 208
neck stiffness 35
Neocon 226
Neogest 227
neomycin 211
neoplasms 110, 111
nerve
  damage 43—4
  impulse transmission 205
neuralgia 221
neural tube defect 172, 224
neuritis 221
neurological symptoms 223
'neurotic symptoms' 26, 27, 45, 55,
        107
New England Journal of Medicine
        146
nicotinamide (aka niacin, B_3) 222
nitrogen 204

noise, sensitivity to 221
nonesterified free fatty acids 209
nonoxynol 188
non-specific genital infections 173, 174—6
non-specific urethritis 189
Nora, J.J. 166
noradrenaline 213
norethisterone 34, 35, 125, 209, 226, 228
  acetate 32, 34, 124—6, 210, 226, 228
norethynodrel 43, 227
Norgeston 227
norgestrel 32, 34, 54, 55, 65, 66, 125, 209, 210, 228
Noriday 226
Norimin 226
Norinyl 34, 226, 227
Norlestrin 226, 228
normal adrenal hormones 203—14
nortestosterones 28—9
Not All in the Mind 85, 86
nuclear fall-out 164
numbness in feet 54
Nuremberg trial 169
nutrition 100, 180—1, 203—25
  of infants 157—63, 172, 219
nystatin 100, 101

Oberlees, Prof. Donald 163
obesity 62, 67, 89, 205
obstetrician 233
oedema 89
Oenothera biennis see evening primrose oil
oestradiol 229, 233
  valerate 229
oestriol 229
oestrogen 17—21, 24—5, 28—37, 40, 41, 51—5, 58—67, 98, 100, 103, 111, 115—17, 122, 124, 129, 130, 132, 134—6, 139—47, 152—5, 157, 166, 169, 170, 177, 182, 191—3, 195, 204, 207, 209—17, 221—2, 225, 227—9, 233
  catechol 52
  conjugated 139, 140, 229, 231
  'natural' 39, 80
oestrogenic moulds 84, 136
oestrogenic mycotoxins 102, 136, 218
oestrone 229
older women
  barrier methods for 199
  and cancer 129—32, 135, 137, 138
  and hormones 143—4
  and oestrogen 103
  and osteoporosis 144—9
Ollier, Dr Bill 91
optic neuritis 43
oral contraceptives 233
  see also pill, the
Oral Contraceptive Advisory Group 22
oranges 74, 86, 88—90
Orlest 226
Ortho Dienoestrol 229
OrthoNovin 226, 227
Ortho-Novum 34, 226
Ory, Dr Howard 132
osteoporosis 63, 67, 143—50, 205, 233
ovarian cancers 129—36, 142, 149—50
ovarian cysts 133, 136, 184
ovarian disease 140, 147, 184, 202
ovariectomies 136, 139—40, 143, 147, 148
ovaries 101, 114, 135—6, 143, 168, 180, 198, 203, 204, 233
overdose
  drug 56
  vitamin 222
overgrowth of womb lining 31, 33
Ovestin 229
Ovran 34, 227
Ovranette 227

ovulation 19—20, 30, 181, 184, 191—3, 233
  Billings method of birth control 191—2
  prevention of 23, 32, 114, 136, 156, 206
Ovulen 34, 227
Ovysmen 226
Oxford/FPA study 45, 72—3, 105, 110, 111, 120, 122, 126, 165, 175—6, 188
oxidation 171
oxygen 70
oxytocin 154

Paffenbarger Dr Ralph 137
pain 206, 225
pancreas 233
papilloedema 43
papilloma virus (type 16) 121, 177
paralysis 34, 42, 43
parents, of girls on pill 198
Park Prewett Hospital 85
pathology 233
Patients' Association 120
Peacock M. 147
peas 89
pelvic inflammatory disease (PID) 129, 130, 132, 133, 147, 174—6, 180, 187, 189
pelvic peritoneal adhesions 175
penicillin 173
penis, deformed 220
Pentovis 229
Pepys, Prof. Jack 90
perinatal deaths 158
periods 30, 198
  heavy see menorrhagia
  and HRT 144
  nerviness during 99
  painful 38, 89, 114
  problems 101, 104
  scanty 54
  see also menstrual; menstruation
pessaries 25, 68, 190

pesticides 102, 225
petrochemicals 92
Pfeiffer, Prof. C.C. 95, 215
pharmacology 233
phenylethylamine 49
phlebitis, venous 38, 98, 234
phytohaemagglutinin (PHA) 98
Pike, Prof. Malcolm 122—5, 137
pill, the
  and allergies 77—102
  body chemistry and 203—25
  and cancer 115—51; see also cancer
  changes in 207
  cost of 200—2
  definiton 233
  future alternatives 186—202
  and metabolic upsets 61—7
  and nutrition 203—25
  side effects of 26—40, 41—60, 200
  and smoking 68—76
  trade names 226—9
  trials 14—15, 16—19, 23—60, 103—40; see also studies and trials
  and young people 152—85
Pill on Trial 106
Pill Victims Group 113
Pincus, Dr Gregory 19, 22
piperazine oestrone sulphate 229
pitocin 154
pituitary 233
  cancer 142
  gland 63, 67, 203, 206, 230
  hormones 154, 197, 204
  tumours 113, 148, 156
placenta 57, 162, 167, 183, 233
platelets 36—7, 75, 80, 95, 205, 225, 233
pleurisy 106, 175
pneumonia 178, 179
poisoning
  accidental 59
  self- 45, 58—9
pollution 77, 93, 144, 164, 167

polycystic ovary disease 66
population control 22—4, 199—200
post-partum depression 55, 57, 59, 80, 215
potassium 206
  bicarbonate 86—7
  ions 205
potency, male 195
prednisone 43, 85, 87, 88, 137, 144, 205, 233
pre-eclampsia 215
pregnancy 18, 143, 203
  and alcoholism 94
  and allergy 80, 81, 91—2
  and cancer 126—7, 134, 152—6
  and congenital abnormality 165—70
  and diaphragm 190
  drugs and 101
  early sickness 80
  ectopic 128, 133, 156, 175—7, 187
  and hormones 20—1, 57, 79, 80, 152—7, 164—73, 184—5, 187, 205
  incidental 126
  increased risk 51, 126, 129, 184
  and IUDs 187, 188
  and low doses 55, 65
  miscarriage and 170
  multiple STD in 179
  and 'natural' birth control 191, 193
  osteoporosis in 148
  and pill 23, 25, 26, 33, 115, 117, 125, 128, 207, 209, 211, 214—16, 218, 219, 221, 225
  and sheath 189
  and sterilisation 196
  supplements for 95
  teenagers and 170, 185, 198
  tests 165
  tubal 174
  unplanned 32, 108, 129, 188, 199
  vaccination against 196—7

vaginal infection and 100, 174
viral infection in 178
vitamins and 219, 222—4
zinc in 161—4, 181—5
Premarin 229, 233
premature labour 156
premature low birth weight babies 162
premenstrual 233
  syndrome (PMS) 18, 30, 47—8, 55, 89, 95, 108, 116, 171, 203
    increased by pill 30, 48, 59, 101
    reduced by pill 26, 29, 45, 48
Prempak 228
prenatal infections 178
Primolut N 228
Princess Margaret Migraine Clinic 68—70
progesterone 17—18, 20—1, 30—1, 52, 63, 65, 80, 100, 116, 139, 141—3, 145, 155, 166, 170, 177, 188, 192, 203, 204, 209, 221, 228—9, 233
progestins 18, 19
progestogens 18, 19, 23—5, 28—36, 40, 44, 46, 50—2, 54—5, 59, 61—6, 75, 80—1, 97, 100, 108, 114—18, 122—5, 127—9, 134, 139—42, 144, 147—8, 154—5, 188, 195—6, 206—7, 209—13, 216—17, 226—9, 233
Progynova 229
prolactin 140—1, 148
prolactinomas 148, 156
promiscuity 170, 185—7, 197
prostaglandins (PGEs) 67, 94—5, 154, 233
prostate 233
protein(s) 61, 63, 83, 144
  metabolism 64—5, 67, 92, 94, 203—4, 211—12, 214, 216, 218—19, 223, 230

plasma 167, 171
Provera 229
pruritis 175
Pryse-Davies, Dr John 50, 153—4
psychiatrist 233
psychological
  dependence 78
  tests 159
psychosis 59, 205, 215, 233
puberty 63
pulmonary artery, thickening of 38
pulmonary embolism 37, 233
pyridoxine (B_6) 212—13, 222, 234

Queen Charlotte's Maternity Hospital 54
quinacrine hydrochloride 188
quinestradol 229
quinestrol 229

Radcliffe Infirmary 196
Rakusen, Jill 127
Randolph, Dr Theron 84—7, 137
Rapp, Dr Doris 100
Rea, Dr Bill 98
relationships
  loving 193—4
  problems with 57—8
relatives, lack of caring 55
reliability of pill 46
renin 206, 234
reproductive organ cancers 115, 129—32, 136
research and development 200—2
respiratory infections 82, 175, 179
Responsible Society 199
retinol 219
rhinitis 81, 175
  allergic 106
rhythm method of birth control 190
riboflavin see vitamin B_2
Rice-Wray, Dr Edris 28
Riches, Valerie 198—9
Rimland, Dr Bernard 163—4
RNA 216, 223

Robinson, Jean 120, 127
Robertson, W.F. 166—7
Rock, Dr John 19
Rodrigues, Dr Carmen 170
Roman method (aka coitus interruptus: withdrawal method) 199, 200
Rose, Dr David 212
Rose, Dr Frank Clifford 69
rotation diets 84, 86—90, 102, 113
Rowe, Dr Albert 84
Royal College of General Practitioners 57, 59
  oral contraceptive study report 98, 105—14, 116, 118, 120, 126, 165, 175, 210
Royal College of Physicians 157
Royal Society of Medicine 170
Royal Surrey County Hospital 69, 81, 83, 213—14
Royal Veterinary College 84, 136
Russia, contraception in 199

'safe' periods 193
safety of pills, trials to evaluate 103—14, 125, 196—200, 202
St Mary's Hospital, Paddington 44, 207, 212
saliva 178, 179
salpingitis (infected tubes) 156, 176, 187, 188
salt — water
  balance 63, 67
  metabolism 206, 230
Sandler, Prof. Merton 50, 51
Sanger, Margaret 22
sarcoma 116—17, 234
'Saying No' (handbook) 199
Schering (German firm) 18
schizophrenia 53, 59, 60, 106—7, 164, 205, 215, 216, 234
Schizophrenia Association of Great Britain 59
Schoental, Dr Regina 84, 136, 154, 155, 170

Scholastic Aptitude Test (SAT) 163—4
schoolgirls on pill 197—8
  see also young girls
Selby, P.L. 147
selenium 218
self-injury 45
self-poisoning 45, 58
Selye, Hans 75
semen 94
  abnormalities 156
  AIDS virus 179
seminal fluid 190
Sequens 228
sequential pills 31—3, 41, 51, 52, 54, 104, 116, 226—9, 234
serotonin 156, 212—13, 234
Sex and Destiny 199
sex hormone(s) 203, 220
  dependent cancers 129—32
sexual desire *see* libido
sexual development, precocious 170, 185—7
sexual dysfunction 67
sexual intercourse
  abstention from 190—4
  as act of trust 199
  painful *see* dyspareunia
sexually transmitted diseases (STD, orig. VD) 120—2, 143, 173—9, 185, 189, 199
sexual organ abnormalities 117, 135, 149, 154—5
sheaths, contraceptive 25, 68, 188, 189, 199
sick leave 47—8
side effects, and pill 200
  as 'neurotic symptoms' 26—7, 45, 55, 107
  reduction of 29
  in trials 26—40, 41—60
Singer, Dr Albert 121
sinusitis 175
sinusoids 234
  dilated endometrial 35—7

Sjögren's syndrome 148
skin
  birthmarks 170
  healthy 220
  pigmented 56
  rashes 81, 86, 96, 99
slurred speech 43
Smith, Dr George 152
Smith, Olive 152
Smuthells, Prof. R.W. 172, 224
smoking 15, 39, 59, 64, 68—76, 78, 83, 85, 87—90, 92—3, 96, 109, 111, 113, 120, 143—4, 158, 164—5, 167, 169, 171—2, 177, 181, 186, 201, 211, 215—16, 222—3, 225
social class 69, 112, 120, 123, 142, 172, 189, 218, 219, 224
social costs of pill 201
social reasons for violence to children 55—6
Society for the Study of Fertility 27
sodium 206
  bicarbonate 86—7
  ions 205
sore leg veins 28, 35, 40, 62
Spellacy Prof. William 125, 209
sperm
  counts 195
  defects 180—1, 202
  production 19, 20, 80, 120, 187, 189, 190, 192, 193
spermicides 189, 190, 199
spina bifida 166, 171, 223
spinal cord, degeneration of 225
sponge caps 190, 196
sprays 196
squint 167
starvation 168
STD *see* sexually transmitted diseases
sterilisation 68, 169, 188, 195—7
sterility 156, 174, 175, 198, 221
Sterns, Gerald 113
steroid(s) 234

hormones *passim*; *see also* pill, the

withdrawal 57, 59, 106—7

stiffness 221

stilboestrol 127, 136, 140—1, 152—4, 156, 157, 170, 229, 234

stillbirth 156, 158—9, 162, 167, 179, 181, 221

stimulants 96

stress 17, 29, 63, 64, 67, 75, 93, 144, 148, 150, 168, 205, 206, 210, 218, 223

strokes 34, 43, 106, 113, 196
    haemorrhagic 109
    thrombolic 109

stromal condensation 37, 234

studies and trials, of pill 14—15, 16—19, 23—60, 103—40
    Atlanta Centers for Disease Control 127, 132—5
    Baltimore 179
    Framingham Heart Study 146—7
    Harvard 146, 147
    Israeli 184
    Jerusalem 128, 170
    London Trials 14, 22—60, 61, 125
    MRC 182
    Oxford/FPA 45, 72—3, 105, 110, 111, 120, 122, 126, 165, 175—6, 188
    Puerto Rico 169—70
    RCGP 98, 105—14, 116, 118, 120, 126, 165, 175, 210
    St Mary's 207—8
    Walnut Creek 58—9, 72—3, 103—4, 110—11, 120, 129—33, 136, 140, 147, 175, 216
    WHO 193

subarachnoid haemorrhage 39, 109, 234

sub-fertility 195

subnuclear vacuoles 31, 125

sugar 100, 174, 182, 218
    cane 89, 223
    craving for 217

sugars (body) 204, 205, 223

suicide 45—7, 53, 56—9, 92, 96—7, 107, 109—10, 113, 172, 212

Sunday Times 176

sunlight, reactions to 99, 222

superficial phlebitis 234

Suporn, Dr 128

suppositories 228

Surrey University 214

sweat(ing) 143
    analysis tests 160—1, 180—1, 183, 185, 217, 218

Swedish Regulatory Board 66

Swyer, Dr Gerald 14, 26, 124

sympto-thermal method of birth control 193

Syntex ('US) 18

syphilis 173, 174, 177

talcum powder 135

tampons 190

Tampovagan 229

taste
    poor sense of 216
    test, zinc 183—5

tea 86, 89, 93, 211

teenagers on pill 176

teeth, healthy 220

temperature checks 191—3

temporary suppression of symptoms 114

tension 46, 71, 73
    premenstrual *see* premenstrual syndrome

teratogens 166, 167

testes 203, 204, 234
    abnormal 117, 155, 156, 184, 202, 220

testicular cancer 117, 135, 142, 155, 156, 184

testosterone 18, 65—6, 117, 141, 155, 195, 204, 206, 226—8, 234
test-tube babies 155
tetracyclines 178, 225
Thailand, University Hospital 128
Thalidomide 166—7, 221
thermometers, electronic 192—3
thiamin *see* vitamin B$_1$
Third World countries 201, 202, 219
Thomas, Dylan 91
throat, dry 148
thromboembolic disease 41, 109, 111
thrombolic stroke 109
thrombo-phlebitis 35, 36, 54, 98
thrombosis 61, 80, 98, 106—7, 124, 217, 225, 227, 234
  episodes 75
  venous 14, 33—44, 56, 141, 169
thrush (candidiasis, aka monilia) 100, 173—5, 220
thyroid
  activity 63, 67, 203
  cancer 111
  extract 38
  hormones 204
  problems 217
thyroxine 217
tiredness 42, 51, 55, 62, 88, 89, 96, 99, 221
tissue
  damage 80
  typing 91
tobacco addiction *see* smoking
tongue
  coated 222
  sore 225
total allergy syndrome 93
toxicity
  chemical 102, 142, 167—8, 225
  metal 100, 120, 144, 148, 151, 158, 160—2, 167—8, 181, 187, 225

toxic-shock syndrome 190
traffic fumes 88, 99, 142, 144
tranquillisers 16, 38, 56, 73, 76, 111
tremors 222
trichomonas vaginalis 100, 175, 179
trichomoniasis 175
tricyclic antidepressants 211
triglycerides 209, 210, 234
Trinordiol 227
Trinovum 226
triphasic 65
Trisequens 228
tryptophan 234
  serotonin pathway 212
tubal blockages 174
tubal damage 174
tubal infections (salpingitis) 156, 176, 187, 188
tuberculosis 48, 211
tumours 80, 111, 116, 117, 152—4, 177, 228
  malignant 128—9
  pituitary 113
Turnbull, Prof. Alex 141
twins 167, 168
tyramine 49
tyrosine 213

ulcerative colitis 106
ulcers
  genital 177—8
  mouth 222
University College Hospital 14, 26
University of California 162
University of Illinois 189
ureaplasma urealyticum 179
urethra, ageing changes in 143
urinary infections 87, 175
urinary pain 88
urinary tract
  cancer 222
  neoplasms 111
urine tests 191, 212
urogenital problems 220
US Air Force 39

US Navy 163
uterine cancer 142
uterine disease 140
uterine fibroids 38
uterine infections 174—5
uterus 234
Utovlan 228

vaccination against pregnancy
    196—7
vacuoles 31—2
vaginal cancer 142, 152—4, 184
vaginal cells 52
vaginal discharge 106—7
vaginal dryness 143, 148
vaginal infections 100, 174
vaginal secretions 52, 100
vaginal smears 25
vaginal thrush 175
vaginitis 175
Valium 73
varicose veins 44, 188
    burst 55
vascular abnormalities 170
vascular accidents 38, 113
vascular cancer of tongue 128
vascular changes 62, 145, 146
vascular disease 15, 39, 68, 69, 70,
    72, 76, 109, 110, 113, 116,
    146, 147, 217
vascular tumour 117
vasculitis 43
vasectomy 196
vasodilation 70
Vaughan, Paul 106
vault cap (vimule) 190
vegetable(s)
    green 224
    oils 171
vegetarians 181, 182, 224
vein(s)
    changes 33, 41, 44, 54, 55, 78
    clots in 34
    distended 32, 35—6, 44
    thrombosis 38, 40, 44

venereal diseases see sexually
    transmitted diseases
venous phlebitis 38
venous thrombosis 14, 33—44, 148,
    208
venous thromboembolic disease 41,
    109, 111
Vessey, Prof. Martin 109—10, 123,
    126
vimule (vault cap) 190
violence 47, 53, 89, 100, 181
    towards children 48, 55—7
    crime and low SAT scores 164
    death by 58—9, 106—7, 110—11
viral infections 98, 107, 117, 225
virus diseases 106
vitamin A 64, 167, 171, 219—20
vitamin B_1 (thiamine) 220—2
vitamin B_2 (riboflavin) 64, 167,
    172, 221, 234
vitamin B_3 (nicotinamide; aka
    niacin) 222
vitamin B_6 (pyridoxene) 64,
    100—1, 172, 212—13, 217,
    222, 234
vitamin B_{12} 64, 167, 172, 223,
    224—5
vitamin B complex 171, 172,
    220—5
vitamin C (ascorbic acid) 64, 67,
    160, 167, 171—2, 211, 223,
    225, 230
vitamin D 144, 148, 151
vitamin E 171
vitamin(s) 63, 120, 167—8, 214,
    218—25
    low allergy pills 101
    supplements 89, 95—6, 100—2,
        148, 158, 162, 172, 183,
        185, 224—5
Volans, Dr Glynn 70
Volidan 228
vomiting 116, 224
vulvar warts 177

Walnut Creek contraceptive study 58—9, 72—3, 103—4, 110—11, 120, 129—33, 136, 140, 147, 175, 216
Walsh, Dr Frank 43
water metabolism 203, 205
Weid, Prof. 32, 118
weight
  gain 27, 32, 43, 54—5, 62—3, 67, 184, 195, 208
  problems 67, 78, 134, 170
Weindling, H. 65
Westminster Hospital Immunology Unit 82
wheat 87, 89, 90, 93, 172, 222—3
Wilkinson, Dr Marcia 69
withdrawal
  method of birth control (coitus interruptus, aka Roman method) 199, 200
  symptoms 78, 87, 95, 106—7, 144
womb
  cancers 116, 147, 150
  changes to arteries 39—40, 44
  changes to veins 35—6, 44
  contraction 203
  disorders 140
  enlarged 42
  lining changes 49—50, 108, 115, 134, 179, 216
    and brain changes 50—2
  protection 190
Women's National Cancer Control Campaign 121
work, sick leave from 47—8
World Health Organisation (WHO) 121, 194, 195
ovulation method study 193
World Medicine 118
Wright, Dr Helen Layling 37, 189
Wynn, Professor Victor 44, 65, 207—10, 212, 213

X-rays 166

Yale University Medical School 196
yeast 86, 87, 89, 93, 100—1, 102, 148, 160, 174, 182, 216, 218, 220—3, 225
young girls on pill 63, 101, 184, 225
  advice to 197—200
  anorexia in 92, 148, 183—4, 224
  and cervical cancer 118—19
  with osteoporosis 148
  precocious sexual development in 170, 185—7
  pregnant 152
  STD and 173, 179
  as targets for cancer 142—3
  vaginal cancer in 152

zeralenone 170
zeranol 170
zinc 57, 60, 64—6, 95, 100, 120, 144—6, 148, 151, 158—65, 167, 171—2, 180—5, 213—17, 219, 223—4, 230, 234
  sulphate 180, 183—4
  taste test 183—4
zona pellucida 197